HOW TO LIVE TO BE
100
YEARS OLD

GARRY GORDON

BALBOA.
PRESS

A DIVISION OF HAY HOUSE

Balboa Press books may be ordered through booksellers or by contacting:

Balboa Press
A Division of Hay House
1663 Liberty Drive
Bloomington, IN 47403
www.balboapress.com.au
1 (877) 407-4847

Print information available on the last page.

ISBN: 978-1-5043-1581-4 (sc)
ISBN: 978-1-5043-1592-0 (e)

Balboa Press rev. date: 11/14/2018

When the student is ready
the teacher will appear.

ACKNOWLEDGEMENTS

During my journey to climb Mt Everest in the form of this book, there were many people who inspired me and helped me along the way. I would like to thank those who have inspired me the most:

- Thank you, God, for the gift of writing
- Thank you, my loving wife
- Thank you, Max, for believing in me
- Thank you, Bruce, for teaching me many life lessons
- Thank you, Father Dennis, for your wisdom
- Thank you, David, for your multi-media expertise
- Thank you to the people who have placed barriers before me in writing this book as you helped me build my character.

Kind Regards

Garry

DEDICATION

To my wife Rose.

I love you. Thank you. The courage you have shown with the struggles in your life is an inspiration.

To the health pioneers who have blazed a trail to help heal many people, you have truly touched my spirit:

- Anne Wigmore – who showed that wheatgrass has amazing healing properties.
- Max Gerson – has cured more people of cancer and major diseases than any other person.
- Louis Hay – mind, body and spirit.

To God, the source of creativity. Thank you for inspiring me with the gift of health.

CONTENTS

INTRODUCTION

Shrouded in mystery, 9000 feet above sea level surrounded by air stirred up from Mt Everest, lies the mystical Shangri La.

Your spirit is soaring to finally, like an eagle, touch down in the "Valley of the Longevity Giants", the Hunza people. There, you will meet the most astonishing people on the face of the planet.

The Hunza people are poor in money and possessions but rich in spirit:

- no sick people to be seen
- no military force
- no shops
- no negative attitudes.

They have:

- abundant health
- abounding happiness
- peace of mind deep in their spirit
- the energy to walk 10 to 20 kilometres
- wisdom to really take care of their families
- a surprising number of their people who live to be 100 years old.

The Hunza people have the ability to be responsible for their own actions and that is why they are careful about what they eat, their exercise habits, e.g. walking and yoga, and maintaining positive thought patterns.

It is time to look into a mirror and face yourself – take a look at your naked self and do not blame anybody or anything else for what you see.

The Hunza people who are legends of longevity have the ability to face themselves and take responsibility for their own actions. One of the mysteries of life is why do we get sick? What are some of the laws or life principles that can literally change our life if we were to embrace them.

Mind, body and spirit

Let us look at this from a mind, body and spirit perspective and face ourselves.

The mind

All of life flows from our thoughts. Emerson, Socrates and others taught these things. All the answers to life are inside of us, they come to the surface during meditation and prayers. It is important to find a quiet place to sit and relax and ask ourselves some important questions. What thoughts have I had that have given me sickness, stress, anxiety, unforgiveness? What new thoughts can I have to transform my life?

The new thoughts we could have for ourselves and towards others are peaceful thoughts, loving thoughts, supportive thoughts, happy thoughts, and forgiving thoughts. Now let us look at the types of negative thoughts we might have towards ourselves and others such as hateful thoughts, criticizing thoughts, fearful thoughts, and revengeful thoughts and actions to others who have wronged us instead of forgiveness.

What you give to yourself and others, you will keep attracting into your life. This is the "Law of Attraction".

The body

What food you feed your body will help give you sickness or abundant health. Too much "acid forming food" like meat and too much fast food full of fat will help create sickness in your body over a period of time. Yes, it is you who contributes to causing the disease in your body, not your mother or father or the clever advertisements about unhealthy foods on TV. The good news is by making better choices like eating more "alkaline forming food" like vegetables, salad and fruit, we can literally transform our lives from the inside to the outside of our bodies, over a period of time.

As our internal awareness grows, we ask ourselves questions like: What breakfast is great for long-term energy, health, vitality and long life? What will be my lunch today to give me more focus, strength, creativity and health? What will be my dinner this evening that will refuel my body giving me more life, peace, energy and endurance?

Healthy food will give you the energy to kick start your body to fire you up to start exercising such as walking 20 minutes three times a week, Tai Chi, yoga, swimming, lifting small weights, golf, tennis etc. Your body needs exercise to get your heart pumping more highly oxygenated blood around your body to nourish all vital organs, reduce stress and anxiety, help remove toxins from the body, help lose weight and fat and to give us a more flexible body full of energy. What exercise can I start today for my health and my family's health? What relaxing exercise can I begin to kick start my life now?

The spirit

What spiritual vitamins can I give myself today? How can I support myself and my family and my friends and my work colleagues? We can give to ourselves by supporting ourselves and give to others by supporting and encouraging other people without thinking about getting anything in return. It is about loving and caring for ourselves and loving and caring for other people, this is different from romantic love for another person. We can choose happiness for ourselves and give happiness to other people.

Living a spiritual life is about being thankful for what you have received rather than complaining too much, because what you focus on will increase in your life. This leads to giving and receiving which is part of the law of increasing returns or the law of diminishing returns. Whatever you give to other people, whether good or bad, will start to increase in your life. This is also known as the law of the farm, that is, when you plant tomato seeds you will harvest tomatoes not watermelons. The law of diminishing returns means whatever you withhold from other people will be withheld from you, such as withholding love or kindness from other people.

Spiritual things involve intuition, creativity, inspiration, truth, healing, compassion, trust and wisdom. In his book, *The Seat of the Soul*, Gary Zukav talks about love, compassion and wisdom. He says they do not come from the personality, instead they are experiences of the soul. Your soul is the part of you that is immortal.

Listen to the wisdom of the ancients
whispering your guidance within.

Whatever you put in your mouth every day over many years will determine your chances of living to be 100 years old like the biblical patriarchs.

You have control over your body. It is better to be master of yourself than the master of an army. To be master of yourself you need to be master of your habits. Either you master your habits or your habits will master you.

Habit

I am your constant companion
I am your greatest helper or heaviest burden
I will push you onward ... or
Drag you down to failure
I am completely at your command
Half the things you do you might just as well turn over to me and I will do them quickly
I am easily managed but you must be firm with me
Show me exactly how you want things done and after a few lessons I will do it automatically
I am the servant of all great people
But also of all failures as well
Those who are failures I have made them failures
Take me, train me, be firm with me and I will put the world at your feet
Be easy with me and I will destroy you
Who am I? I am habit!
The beginning of a habit is like an invisible thread
But every time we repeat the act we strengthen the strand
Add to it another strand until it becomes a great cable
And this cable can become impossible to break
Orison Swett Marsden

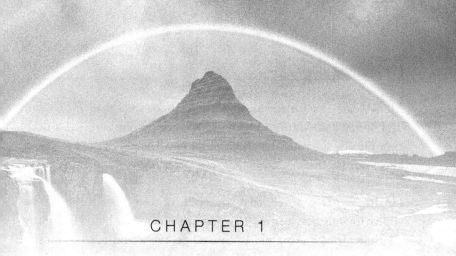

CHAPTER 1

ACID /ALKALINE FOODS

One of the most amazing discoveries of the 21st century besides Neil Armstrong stepping foot onto the moon is that your blood pH should be alkaline between 7.1 to 7.5.

If your blood pH is alkaline this will greatly reduce your chances of suffering a heart attack or contracting cancer. Having alkaline blood will mean an increase in the oxygen in your blood, whereas, if your blood is acidic, a pH of 6.5 to 6.9, the oxygen concentration in your blood will be less.

Cancer loves an acidic environment and what happens generally is the cells start to multiply rapidly in the body at the weakest link, e.g. the liver or stomach etc.

Having a slightly alkaline blood is one of the keys to a long life and that is why the Hunza people, the Okinawa people and people from most other communities with greater longevity eat mostly vegetable and fruits.

My journey

Many years ago I made an important discovery. I read *Fit for Life* by Harvey and Marilyn Diamond and something touched a deep chord inside me when I learned about how the pH of our blood can affect our health.

Health experts agree that the pH of our blood should be approximately between 7.1 to 7.5 which means our blood is slightly alkaline. To achieve a pH in this range, we would need to mostly eat fruits and vegetables. While our blood remains slightly alkaline, it is far more difficult for major diseases to gain a foothold. When our blood is slightly acidic, that is 5.5 to 6.9, this means we are eating too much protein and carbohydrates, which can lead to many diseases. Dr Paavo Airola, a world famous nutritionist, believes that having acidic blood is the basic cause of all disease and acidic blood will result if we don't eat enough alkaline foods to balance the acidic foods we eat over a period of time. One of the consequences of acidic blood is that acid will be deposited in the joints and tissues over many years slowly creating diseases such as arthritis which many people suffer in their later years. Dr Airola's book, *How to Get Well*, published by Health Plus is a valuable reference about acid and alkaline forming foods.

My personal journey into acid and alkaline forming foods began when I discovered that the pH of our saliva closely follows the pH of our blood which meant I could easily and regularly check the pH of my blood by testing my saliva.

This is the method I used to test the pH of my saliva. First, I purchased a packet of pH testing strips. Then, two hours after eating food or fluids I would place the pH paper on my tongue and rub saliva onto the pH paper. I would wait about 15 seconds and then match the colour of the pH paper to the colour printed on the side of the packet as a reference. When I first tested for pH, the colour matched 6.5 which is slightly acidic. This was an "aha" moment where I realised I had been eating mostly meat and potatoes with very little vegetables and fruit in my diet and was not doing much exercise. No wonder I was always tired and fatigued and had little energy.

This was a turning point in my life. It was as if an angel had landed on my shoulder and whispered, "It is time you are at the crossroads of your life. Move forward into an alkaline and healthy life or go backwards into an acidic and sickly life. Change is inevitable."

My journey, during which my blood chemistry changed from acidic to alkaline took three months.

Vitality, energy, a more positive attitude and abundant health began to take roots deep inside me.

Let food be thy medicine. – Hippocrates

How different foods are classified: alkaline forming or acidic forming

The following is an important guide that explains how different foods are classified as to whether they are alkaline forming in the body or acidic forming in the body. It would be wise to achieve greater longevity by eating mostly alkaline forming food, say 80% and 20% acid forming foods.

Food category	High alkaline	Alkaline	Low alkaline	Low acid	Acid	High acid
Vegetables	Barley grass Broccoli Celery Garlic	Green beans Lima beans Beets Carrots Lettuce Zucchini	Asparagus Beetroot Cabbage Fresh corn Cauliflower Mushrooms Onions Olives Potatoes Squash Soybeans Tofu	Cooked spinach Kidney Beans Sweet potatoes	Pinto Beans Navy beans	Pickled vegetables
Fruit	Dried figs Raisins	Apples Berries Black-currants Dates Grapes Kiwi fruit Papaya Pears	Avocados Coconuts Cherries Grapefruit Lemons Mango Oranges Papaya Pineapple Peaches Strawberry Tomatoes Watermelon	Bananas Blueberry Cranberry Plums	Canned fruit	
Grains and Cereals			Amaranth Buckwheat Lentils Millet Quinoa	Brown rice Oats Rye bread Whole grain bread		
Meat				Liver Oysters	Chicken Fish Lamb	Beef Pork Shellfish Sardines
Eggs and Dairy		Breast milk	Goat milk Soya milk	Milk Yogurt	Eggs Hard cheese	
Nuts and seeds		Almonds Hazelnuts	Brazil nuts	Pumpkin seeds	Cashews Pecans	Peanuts Walnuts

Let us follow the wise leaders of the past

Famous vegetarians

- Leonardo de Vinci
- Albert Einstein
- Socrates
- Plato
- St Francis of Assisi
- George Bernard Shaw

Why did the wise leaders of the past eat mostly vegetarian food? Let us examine some facts. Your body is designed of cells. Your cells need energy, vitamins, minerals, protein and water.

What your cells need

Important Vitamins

Vitamin A – For good vision, skin and hair. Food sources: carrots, green leafy vegetables, pumpkin, coloured fruits and vegetables

Vitamin B1 (thiamine) – Very important for the nervous system and digestive system, helps maintain normal red blood count, prevents fatigue and gives greater stamina. Food sources: wheat germ, whole grain cereals, all seeds and nuts, green leafy vegetables and potatoes.

Vitamin B2 (riboflavin) – Essential for general health, eyes, skin, hair and nails. Food sources: milk, cheese, eggs, wheat germ, almonds and sunflower seeds.

Vitamin B3 (niacin) – Important for good circulation, nervous system and intestinal health. Food sources: brown rice, seeds, nuts, green vegetables, wheat germ and rice bran.

Vitamin B5 (pantothenic acid) – Good for the hair and helps increase the action of other B vitamins. Food sources: seeds, grains and brown rice.

Vitamin B6 (pyridoxine) – Helps build enzymes in the body, helps the nervous system, helps the essential balance between potassium and sodium in the body, and contributes towards longevity. Food sources: wheat germ, soya beans, bananas, avocado, walnuts, cabbage, carrots and green peppers.

Vitamin B9 (folic acid) – Needed during pregnancy, functions together with vitamin B12 in many body processes such as cell division. Food sources: most green leafy vegetables, wheat germ, soya beans, kidney beans, lima beans, chickpeas, asparagus, lentils and walnuts.

Vitamin B12 – (cyanocobalamin) – Needed for the generation of red blood cells. Food sources: clams, oysters, sardines, salmon and Swiss cheese.

Vitamin B17 – (nitrilosides) – Helps prevent cancer in the body and discovered by Dr E. Krebs – Food sources – Apricots and particularly the seed kernel, apple seeds.

Vitamin C – Important for wound repair, an essential antioxidant, improves the immune system especially related to colds and flu. Food sources: red peppers, kale, broccoli, Brussels sprouts, oranges and lemons.

Vitamin D – Prevents rickets in the bones, helps prevent tooth decay, helps prevent depression and is also known as the "sunshine vitamin". Food sources: sardines, eggs, mushrooms and sprouted seeds.

Vitamin E – Helps increase the efficiency of the muscular system especially the heart and helps with fertility for men and women.

Food sources: sprouted seeds, fresh wheat germ and green leafy vegetables.

Vitamin F (lecithin) – Lowers blood cholesterol, helps prevent heart disease and important for all glands especially the adrenal glands. Food sources: flaxseed oil, sunflower oil.

Vitamin K – Known as the blood-clotting vitamin and it helps to prevent strokes. Food sources: green leafy vegetables, alfalfa, cabbage and wheat germ.

Vitamin P (rutin) – Helps with high blood pressure and helps with eye diseases. Food sources: buck wheat, blackcurrants, strawberries and cherries.

Important Minerals

Calcium – Essential for building bones and teeth, important when breast feeding, very important for elderly people, helps create and maintain a healthy heart, stimulates the activity of enzymes and assists in controlling the acid / alkaline balance in the body. Food sources: kelp has 1000 mg of calcium per 100 g, cheese, kale, yogurt, almonds, parsley, figs, and milk has 100 mg of calcium per 100 g.

Chlorine – One of the main ingredients in common salt, too much salt in the body causes many health problems, e.g. overweight and high blood pressure. Food sources: salt, eggplant and sweet potato.

Copper – Helps in the development of connective tissues, brain and nerves. Food sources: green leafy vegetables, raisins, pomegranates, beans and peas.

Chromium – Insulin and chromium help remove glucose from the blood, helps the heart and helps in overcoming diabetes. Food sources: mushrooms and whole grain bread.

Iodine – Very important for a healthy thyroid gland. Food sources: kelp and iodised salt.

Iron – Essential for red blood cells, women lose iron during the menstrual period. Food sources: parsley, strawberries and green leafy vegetables.

Magnesium – About 60% of magnesium is found in bones, and it is vitally important for the nervous system. Food sources: kelp, wheat germ, almonds, Brazil nuts, cashew nuts and buckwheat.

Phosphorous – Helps the nervous system, mostly found in bones, and calcium and phosphorous work together. Food sources: yogurt, lentils, salmon, chicken and beef.

Potassium – One of the most important alkaline minerals missing in the diet of most people, potassium and sodium work together to help control body / fluid balance, being an alkaline mineral it helps to balance when there is too much acid in the blood stream, and arthritis and bone problems are the main result or eating too much acid forming food over a long period of time. Food sources: kelp, parsley, apricots and bananas.

Silicon – Helps the body maintain healthy nails, hair and skin. Food sources: lettuce, parsnips, asparagus, horseradish and sunflower seeds.

Sodium – The sodium / potassium ratio in the body is vitally important especially in the kidneys and most people have too much sodium (from salt) and not enough potassium. Food source: salt.

Zinc – Important for fertility especially in men, and helps the prostate gland function efficiently. Food sources: oysters and pumpkin seed kernels.

Hopefully, we have learnt more about what the cells in our body need for optimum health. Now, let us have a look in nature's animal kingdom at how the carnivores and herbivores are designed.

How carnivores and herbivores are designed

How did God design carnivores?

Carnivores (meat eaters) generally have large prominent teeth designed for catching and bringing down their prey. The jaw of a tiger can only move up and down, whereas, human teeth can move side to side exactly like a herbivore (plant eater). A tiger's stomach is basically in a straight line with a bag at the end. The meat comes into the mouth and is not chewed which is very different from our way of eating meat. Tigers eat raw meat while we eat cooked meat because our stomach is not designed to eat raw meat. Our intestines are shaped like multiple S letters and are about seven metres long which is a perfect design to digest fibrous material like plant food while a tiger's intestines are very different from ours. A tiger's tongue is rough and is designed for drinking water from a river or water hole and for licking blood. Human saliva has an enzyme called ptyalin which helps pre-digest carbohydrates like bread and grain foods, whereas, a tiger has no such enzyme in its saliva. A tiger's stomach has 10 times the amount of hydrochloric acid and, therefore, is perfectly designed for digesting meat. In comparison, a human stomach has a much weaker concentration of hydrochloric acid. Furthermore, carnivores generally have a shorter life span than herbivores possibly because of the amount of acid forming meat they eat.

How did God design herbivores?

Herbivores (plant eaters) have teeth designed for chewing their plant-based food from side to side, similar to our way of eating food. Plant eater's intestines are shaped like multiple S letters and are very much different in design to those of a carnivore, for example, our intestines are about seven metres long which is a perfect design for eating plant-based food that needs a lot of digestion. Our tongue is smooth similar to a herbivore's tongue, while a carnivore's tongue is rough. A herbivore's life span is generally greater than a carnivore's life span, for example, the Galapagos tortoise can live to more than 100 years old. Herbivores are peaceful as they eat plant based food, whereas, most carnivores are aggressive as they eat meat. In addition, herbivores have sweat pores for elimination of toxins and when they sweat this allows evaporation for heat control. Furthermore, they do not eat meat that contains cholesterol as all plant-based food have no cholesterol. Herbivores eat plants, which are alkaline forming in their body.

The human body is designed to eat plant based food

The more plant-based food you eat the longer you will live. I often like to compare an acid battery that you would put in a torch with an alkaline battery. The alkaline battery will always last longer than the acid battery. When you consistently eat more alkaline forming foods like vegetables and fruit rather than acid forming foods, you too can live a longer disease-free life like the Hunza people.

In Australia, there was a man who followed the Hunza way of eating. His name is Eric Storm these are the facts:

- Born 4th March 1896 and died 24th February 2000 at the age of 103
- Suffered a heart attack at the age of 34 years old
- His doctor warned him if he did not change he would not live a long life
- Eric Storm started to follow the Hunza way of eating mostly plant-based food which is alkaline forming in the body
- He lived an energetic and active life and passed away aged 103
- Roger French, his close friend, wrote a book called *The man who lived in three centuries.*

What you eat every day will slowly but surely decide your future health. If you eat healthy alkaline forming foods 80% of the time, then you will be pain-free, vibrant, full of energy and the universe will smile on you and you will have a long and happy life. Whereas, if you eat mostly acidic forming foods like too much meat, fatty and processed food, then slowly darkness will descend on your body in the form of sickness, and pain in your joints from the build-up of uric acid. Your emotions will lean to the negative side and you will live a short, painful and unhappy life.

The father of medicine, Hippocrates said, "Let food be thy medicine", and we either learn the wisdom of this brilliant man or we are doomed to eat the wrong types of food and suffer the consequences in the form of painful sickness in our body, such as cancer.

We often eat the wrong types of food because our tongue tempts us and sends messages to our brain to eat more sweet tasting food. There is a constant battle going on inside of us between our tongue and our awareness of what we know in our hearts we should be eating. Who is the boss of what you eat, your tasting tongue or the awareness of what is good for our body?

We are learning the importance of what we eat and the effect of acid and alkaline forming foods which contribute to the pH level of our blood.

Diet and pH levels

What is pH?

pH is a scale which indicates acidity or alkalinity. pH values can range from 1 to 14, where 1 is the most acidic, 14 is the most alkaline and 7 is neutral.

What does pH have to do with us?

Our body's pH levels, e.g. in body fluids like our blood and saliva, are affected by what we eat and drink, along with our general heath and how our organs are functioning. A healthy person will have a blood pH within a narrow range that is slightly alkaline, and a pH outside this range could indicate potential health problems or disease.

The pH of our saliva closely follows the pH of our blood. The pH of our saliva and blood should be in the range of 7.1 to 7.4 which is alkaline. If your pH stays in this range, you are more likely to live a longer life with less disease.

Water is close to neutral with a pH of around 7.0; and the pH of saliva and blood can also be neutral.

When our saliva and blood has a pH of approximately 5.5 to 6.5 this is acidic which will generally mean you are more susceptible to cancer, heart disease, arthritis and many other diseases.

How can our diet affect our pH?

The following table is an experiment where 16 people who I worked with at the time were tested to find the pH levels of their saliva two hours after eating or drinking. Each participant was also asked to describe the food that they normally ate every day. The table clearly shows the more fruit and vegetables eaten by the participant, the more alkaline their saliva and, therefore, the more alkaline their blood will be.

Angela	Breakfast: muesli; average meal: meat and vegetables; plenty of sweet desserts	**7.0** **Neutral**
David	Meat and vegetables, eat meat five times per week; not much fruit	**6.75** **Acidic**
Elsie	Most meals fish & vegetables, sushi, yogurt	**7.25–7.5** **Alkaline**
Garry	Breakfast: green tea, fruit, oats; lunch: salad; dinner: brown rice, fish and plenty of vegetables; 2 pieces fruit per day, 3 dried apricots and 7 apricot kernels per day	**7.25** **Alkaline**

John	Meat and vegetables; past 3 meals had a large portion meat in each meal; one piece of fruit per day	**6.5** **Acidic**
Keith	Meat 3 times per week, fish times a week; 3 pieces of fruit per day	**7.0** **Neutral**
Jay	Breakfast: white/brown rice and vegetables; lunch white/brown rice and vegetables; dinner: brown rice, fish and vegetables	**7.25** **Alkaline**
Lenka	Breakfast: oats, yogurt, wholemeal bread; lunch: chicken and vegetable soup; dinner: pasta with vegetables; not much meat	**7.5** **Alkaline**
Maria	Breakfast: muesli; other meals: mostly vegetables, less meat, not much sweet dessert; apricots and pears every day	**7.5** **Alkaline**
Miles	Meat and vegetables most meals; one piece of fruit per day	**6.5–6.75** **Acidic**
Peter	Breakfast: oats, yogurt; lunch: chicken with green vegetables; dinner: meat twice a week or fish and vegetables normally, sometimes no dinner	**7.5** **Alkaline**
Shirley	Breakfast: oats and toast; meat and vegetables most meals	**7.0** **Neutral**
Segi	No breakfast; meat and chicken with some vegetables; yogurt	**6.75** **Acidic**
Sohel	Rice curries; eat meat once a week, fish and vegetables mostly; one apple per day	**7.25** **Alkaline**
Susana H	Chicken and vegetables mostly with white rice; mandarin and lemon	**7.0** **Neutral**
Susana T	No breakfast; lunch: white rice and vegetables with tofu or noodles; dinner: green tea, white rice, noodles, chips and vegetables; apple, mango and kiwi fruit	**7.25** **Alkaline**
	Date of test week ending 4/7/2011	

One of the best ways to get more alkaline forming foods into our body is by juicing the food we eat.

Juicing

Want to boost your energy levels?

Invest in a good quality juicing machine, e.g. Nutra bullet, Ninja or a simple juice fountain. Severe diseases like cancer, liver problems, heart disease and colon problems have been defeated by juice therapy.

Max Gerson is one of my "health heroes" in using juice therapy to overcome cancer. In the early days, Max suffered severe migraine headaches and his family had a history of migraines. He did research on himself and he tried drinking more milk but he became even sicker. He tried apples and other fruit and his migraines disappeared. After this revelation he stayed on a fruit and vegetable diet for the remainder of his life. Another patient came to Max Gerson suffering from lupus, which even today it is an incurable disease, and Max put this young man on a strict apple diet and he was cured by this treatment.

Max Gerson believed the starting point for many diseases was an imbalance of the potassium/sodium levels in the blood: too much sodium and not enough potassium. We tend to eat far too much salt and processed foods which contain hidden salt levels (sodium). Ask yourself, do you eat too much salt rich food and not enough potassium rich food such as spinach, parsley, kale and most green vegetables?

Too much salt rich processed food and not enough green "potassium charged" food will result over a long period of time in disease such as cancer, high blood pressure, or kidney disease. You have been warned: the decisions you make today about what you eat today will have a huge impact on your life expectancy. Eat mostly fruit and raw vegetables and you could easily live to be 100 years old but eat mostly processed foods from a packet or a can and your life limit could be in your sixties with a strong possibility of many painful years suffering bad health and an early death. If you won't invest in eating healthy foods for your own future, then do it for your wife or husband and children who will be left behind when you die an early death.

Who will take care of your family when you die prematurely? Is it time to change your eating habits so you can love and support your family and teach your children not to follow your bad eating habits? Choose wisely the foods you eat as they are deciding your longevity or early death.

When you are out of the house choose a quality place to buy your juice such as Boost Juice Bars. The founder and managing director, Janine Allis, is a busy working mum and she is a great example of healthy eating and living. I love her company vision: "Every customer who leaves a Boost Juice Bar, will leave feeling that little bit better". When I find myself in a large shopping centre, particularly in the morning or late afternoon, I make the wise choice of, for example, a carrot juice from a Boost Juice Bar to give me a boost of energy that will last me until lunch or dinner. If there is no Boost Juice Bar try Top Juice another quality company. When you choose highly processed foods like donuts, the "sugar hit" only lasts a short time and has no long term positive effect on your health and your life.

In the long term, juice therapy has cured more people of major diseases such as cancer than chemotherapy. For more information, carefully study Max Gerson's life, read Sandra Cabot's books about detoxing the body and read Anne Wigmore's books.

Dr Norman Walker lived to be 114 years old and was a great advocate of juices, for example, carrot juice, and eating raw foods. His book *Becoming Younger* will inspire you to change your eating habits because he proved it by being fit and healthy until the end of his days.

The book *The Man Who Lived in Three Centuries* is about Eric Storm of Australia who lived to be 103 years old and ate mostly raw vegetables and salad. He had a heart attack at 34 years old and it was this event that set his life on the path of healthy unprocessed food. He was living proof that changing your eating habits can change your life so you can live to be a healthy and vibrant 100 year old.

Let us look at the history of a culture, the Hunza people, who mostly eat alkaline forming food.

History of the Hunza Valley discovery

In the late 1920s in India, Major-General Sir Robert McCarrison, then a lieutenant-colonel and physician in the Indian Medical Service, who had spent many years travelling around the Himalayan mountains came across the Hunza Valley. He was astonished to discover the amazing lifespan of the Hunza people who routinely lived 100 to 120 years in this mystical Shangri La.

In addition, Dr McCarrison could not find any evidence of cancer, heart disease, diabetes or degenerative diseases such as arthritis which are common in countries like the USA and Australia. He committed himself to uncovering the extraordinary secrets of the "Fountain of Youth" in the Hunza Valley.

A fateful event occurred in 1927 when he was appointed Director of Nutrition Research in India. God must have been smiling upon him as he was given suitably qualified assistants and a laboratory to carry out experiments. Dr McCarrison was most interested in discovering the role played by the food eaten by the Hunza people in regard to their amazing long lifespans.

Initially, he experimented with over 1000 rats, by feeding them the food normally eaten by the Hunza people, e.g. flat bread made from wholemeal, buckwheat and millet grains, sprouted seeds, raw carrots and cabbage and unpasteurized milk. Like the Hunza people, once a week the rats were fed a small amount of meat. Plentiful water was available in the experiment but no apricots or fruit was given.

For 27 months, the rats were fed the Hunza food and then they were killed and their bodies examined for disease. A stunning discovery was made – no evidence of disease could be found in their bodies.

Why is this amazing knowledge not known widely in the western world?

This is the equivalent of the discovery of the electric light bulb by Thomas Edison and I hope the light of knowledge that shines on you today from Dr McCarrison's experiment will make you think about the importance of eating dynamic healthy food every day.

Let food be your medicine. – Hippocrates.

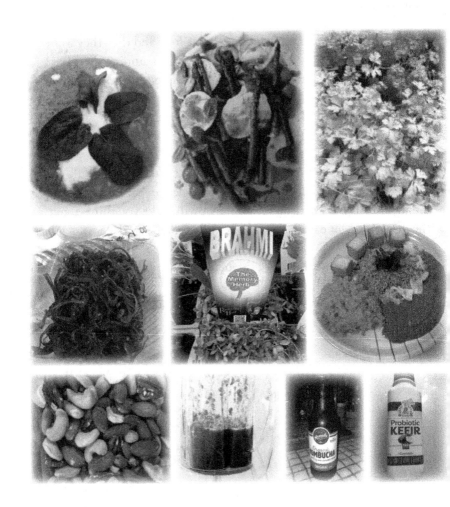

10 Amazing foods to heal your body

1. **Wheatgrass juice.** Ann Wigmore, a pioneer in the use of wheatgrass juice, is one of the health pioneers in the world who I most admire. This juice has healed so many people of major diseases. Please read her book *Be Your Own Doctor*. I have a very personal testimony about wheatgrass juice. Many years ago, my wife was diagnosed with lupus, an incurable disease of the immune system. This was one of the events that triggered my interest in natural medicine. After much research, we tried wheatgrass juice freshly delivered to our door every couple of days. The dose was 30 ml twice a day and after many weeks, a follow-up blood test showed that my wife was cured of lupus. Thank you god for a miracle healing.

2. **Spirulina.** The American space agency NASA has decided this "superfood" will be used by astronauts.

3. **Turmeric.** Indian people eat turmeric in the meals every day and amazingly they have the honour of having the lowest level of Alzheimer's disease in the world.

4. **Dandelion root tea.** The liver is one of the most neglected organs in the body. It is also greatly affected by excessive alcohol consumption. This astonishing organ filters the body of toxins and if your food contains pesticides or toxic chemicals and these get into the bloodstream, your liver will suffer. Dandelion tea has been used for hundreds of years in Germany and other European countries. This tea is one of the best detox treatments you can take into your body.

5. **Goji berries.** These berries are very high in antioxidants.

6. **Deep sea kelp.** The Okinawa people from Japan is a culture with one of the most centenarians in the world. One of their secrets is consuming about 3–4 grams of kelp every day. Kelp has iodine which is good for the thyroid gland and it is full of vitamins and minerals. The great naturopath, Dorothy Hall used kelp on her patients when other treatments did

not work. She said, "There are trace elements in kelp that are sometimes missing from the body" and that can help heal the body from some kinds of disease.

7. **Beetroot/carrot/apple juice.** Max Gerson used this combination of juices to heal cancer and other diseases. Please try it, even after drinking one glass you will feel an uplift in energy levels.
8. **Kefir.** This is fermented drink made from fermented grain used in Europe, the Balkans and in parts of the Middle East. It is similar to Yakult that you can buy in the supermarket. But kefir has less sugar and more good bacteria than other similar products.
9. **Sprouts.** Sprouted seeds are high in enzymes which the body lacks especially as we grow older. Sprouts have levels of B vitamins which help us overcome stress and definitely allows us to sleep better.
10. **Kale.** Kale contains one of the highest levels of antioxidants that help prevent "rust" forming in our blood and keeps us younger inside and outside.

ACT   Action Creates Transformation

Start a health diary to monitor your diet and pH levels and watch how your body's pH changes over time as you modify your diet.

1. Buy some pH papers/strips, e.g. from Alkaway, to test and monitor your blood pH.
2. Two hours after eating or drinking, place a pH paper in your mouth and coat the coloured part of the paper with your saliva. The best time to do this is when you get up in the morning before eating or drinking.
3. Record the colour on the pH paper that matches the guide on the bottle or packet, e.g. 6.5.
4. Buy a small exercise book and write "HEALTH DIARY" on the cover.

5. Every Friday record your pH in a table. Record what types of food you ate during the week. If you can slowly introduce more alkaline foods on a daily basis, your pH will move slowly up to the alkaline range of 7.1 to 7.5. This could take about three months. During this process, there could be days when you feel uncomfortable and this is because the acid toxins are slowly coming out of your body, e.g. via urine, faeces or through your skin.

6. The purpose of this process is to achieve abundant health slowly. As our food habits change, a subsequent change in our vitality and energy levels will be felt as an uplifting experience.

7. Never give up on your dream of a LONG HEALTHY AND ENERGETIC LIFE.

**The Hunza people can do it and I pray that
you can do it too. Have faith!**

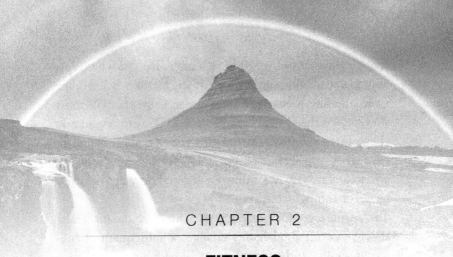

CHAPTER 2

FITNESS

When you were born into this world, the first thing you did was to take your first breath of air. You screamed as the nurse smacked you, resulting in your first gasp of fresh air on this planet.

Your future destiny is that, someday, you will take your last breath.

The purpose of this book is to change your habits to increase your life expectancy to that magic 100 years just like the "Longevity Giants" who live in the Hunza valley.

The Hunza people exercise by walking, yoga, breathing exercises and, believe it or not, playing polo.

Walking habit

As a baby, you first started to crawl and after much trial error you then started to walk. As you grew older you would only start running if someone was chasing you or you were late for a class or an appointment. Walking is your birthright. Driving a car has made us all a little lazy. We are not exercising our muscles when we are driving.

Everything in life is a habit and we all have good habits and bad habits. I would like to take the opportunity to inspire you today to start walking more often starting today. When you are at work, start walking up the stairs instead of using the lift. That is what I do and I can feel my heart pumping when I walk up the stairs to the fifth floor.

Walking is a natural activity that helps the body's lymphatic system. It brings more oxygen into your body, gets your heart pumping and helps with the circulation of your blood. God gave you a healthy body at birth. It is the "temple of the spirit". When you program yourself to make walking a habit, you will notice a big increase in your energy level over about three months.

The walking habit starts today. I am trying to inspire you right now to kick start the walking habit as it will greatly increase the chances of you living to be 100 years old like the Hunza people who have no cars, buses and trains. I believe you can do it.

Benefits of walking

- Results in abundant energy
- Aerobic exercise that introduces more oxygen into your blood, producing alkaline blood
- Greatly reduces stress
- Clears your head when you have problems
- You feel more sexy
- You will lose weight
- One of the best exercises to keep your heart alive and your blood circulating
- Releases tension in your body.

Problems with walking

- If you don't walk enough you will die sooner.

What is stopping you from putting down this book now and opening your front door and walking for 20 minutes?

I DARE YOU ... BECAUSE WHO DARES WINS (SAS commando saying).

Famous walkers and cultures with great longevity

- Jesus Christ as in His day there were no buses, trains or aeroplanes.
- As at 15/8/2013, there was a 123-year-old Bolivian man named Musk who believes a lot of walking is one of the keys to a long and healthy life
- Hunza people are one of the most long lived people groups on the planet
- Okinawa people from Japan who have a long history of centenarians
- Vilcabamba people from Ecuador in South America who have many people living to 100 years plus.

Aerobic exercise

Aerobic exercise is when the heart delivers more oxygen into the muscles for energy production such as when you are walking, swimming, riding a bike, playing tennis, golf or rowing.

Question: What are you doing today to get more oxygen in your body?

- Walking is the simplest exercise to give your body more life sustaining oxygen.
- Eating alkaline food, e.g. fruit and vegetables gives your body more oxygen.
- Diaphragm breathing increases the oxygen in your blood.

- Deep breathing gives you more vitality, dynamic energy and increases the precious oxygen supply in your body.

Almost every day, I walk for at least 20 minutes while breathing deeply through my diaphragm. Some people call this "belly breathing" because you breathe in through your belly not the top of the chest. After walking I can actually feel the increase in dynamic energy by about 20%. When was the last time you felt an increase in your energy levels?

Everyday opportunities for fitness

Climb a mountain or if you can't find a mountain then challenge yourself by walking up a steep hill. When you are at work choose the stairs not the lift, you will feel your heart pumping as you stride higher up the stairs. Your lungs will be expanding with oxygen and you could be sweating as the toxins are coming out of your body. Start slowly for a week and if your fitness level is low only climb one flight of stairs. Every exercise decision you make is increasing your life or decreasing it. In the morning, kick start your day with some exhilarating exercise.

- Stretching is an ideal way to loosen those stiff muscles. Place one hand over the other and stretch your hands above your head. You might hear a clicking sound in your wrist or shoulder as the muscles relax. Do this for ten repetitions.
- Put your hands behind your back and place one hand over the other and stretch downwards. Do this for ten repetitions.
- Extend your hands above your head and rotate your hands backwards about your shoulder for 10 repetitions. Do the same but now rotate your hands forward for ten repetitions. This will relax your shoulders and scapula where stress is often stored.
- With your hands by your side, rotate your shoulders backwards. You will hear a crunching sound but this is

normal. Do this for ten repetitions. Now rotate your shoulders forward. Do this for ten repetitions.

- Your neck is one of the weakest muscles in your body and often gets stiff because you are gazing at a computer screen with your head tilted down slightly. Often, we get tension in our necks from incorrect posture and also emotional issues can cause tension in our neck. A simple exercise to relieve this is to move your head to the right to about 120 degrees only enough that it does not hurt then move your head to the front. Then move your head to the left to about 120 degrees and then move your head to the front again. Do this for ten repetitions on both sides. Turn your head only far enough on each side so it is still comfortable. This is very relaxing for the neck muscles.
- This is good for the lower back. Put your hands on your hips and rotate your hips in a clockwise direction. Do this for ten repetitions. With your hands on your hips now rotate your hips in an anti-clockwise direction. Do this for ten repetitions.

Stretching your muscles at the start of the day will help to energize you and give you extra vitality for your working day.

Journey to work

If you catch the train to work, why not park your car a little further from the railway station and benefit from walking that extra distance to the station. Remember, walking gives you energy. You may need a little extra energy in your working day.

Solar energy power produces Vitamin D

Spend your lunch time walking for 10–15 minutes in the sun. Your bones are getting stronger as your body produces vitamin D, which combines with calcium to boost the strength of your bones like the steel structure of a building.

Lifting small weights

Losing muscle tone and strength can become a problem as we get older. We need to invest in some small dumbbell weights, such as 1 to 2 kg to start with. Do some simple curls with ten repetitions. Lift the weights above your head for ten repetitions. Use your imagination to create a simple exercise program for 10 to 15 minutes per day. Remember, "move or lose it".

Posture

Your body is with you for the rest of your life. How you hold your body and walk with your body can be the cause of pain in your back. How you hold your body is a habit and if you have a sore back from poor posture it will take some time to correct your back. When you are at work sitting in front of a computer all day, how do you align your body to the computer?

Your eyes should be level with the top of the screen. Change the height of the screen if necessary to achieve this. Adjust your chair so your back is straight and your back should be slightly curved. I was talking to a massage therapist who said the fastest growing group of people needing treatment for neck, shoulder and back problems are the 18–25 year olds as a result of poor posture using computers over a period of time. If you would like some proof how posture affects your back, walk down a busy street and notice how many senior citizens over 65 have rounded backs with their chin and head pointed down slightly. Posture affects you eventually as you age. Create good posture now in your life to save yourself from pain in the future. When walking, if you keep your eyes forward, chin in, chest out and stomach in, you are creating a better future for your posture and the longevity of your body. Every change in habit we sustain is helping us live a longer life.

An ideal day in your life

An ideal day could be getting eight hours sleep, eating a healthy breakfast, walking in the morning or evening, being happy at work and finding ways to inspire and help people. The more you inspire and help people the happier you will become. When you arrive home, kiss and hug your partner. Your relationship with your partner and children is important for you and your future. The atmosphere you have at home of joy, trust and love is something you create every day. Life will have problems and struggles at times and developing a positive attitude will change the way we see problems. We start to see problems as a way to change our character to develop persistence, tolerance, patience and compassion. When we look back at problems in life we often find they lead us to a better way of life or we change in some way that is better for our future.

Exploring nature

The Hunza people of northern Pakistan, many of whom live to be 100 years old, walk to their orchards every day with breath taking scenery along the way. There is something about walking in nature, breathing in deeply the vibrant air and listening to the birds chirping in the distant trees that eases our stresses in life and lessens our worries and burdens. In western society, it is often on the weekends that the possibilities open up to us like an oyster revealing the pearl inside. To travel in the country and explore the countryside.

In Sydney, amazing places like the Blue Mountains allow us to get out of our cars and be touched by nature. We can put on our comfortable walking shoes and explore the many walking tracks, ensuring we have a hat to protect us from the sun and sufficient water and food with us. Walking in nature amongst trees and flowers with the smell of the bush engages our senses making us feel more alive and vibrant. As we walk in the bush or even on the side of the road, our hearts are pumping, our circulation is improving and our lungs are expanding. We need this contact with all the elements of nature to relax us and stimulate our senses. For the Aboriginal people who lead a nomadic life in the bush, the longer they spend in the bush the sharper their senses become and the greater their awareness becomes of the plants, the native animals and birds. Similarly, spending time in the country helps renew our internal spirit, away from the noise of computers, cars and city life. We instinctively know we need to spend some time with nature to reduce stress in life and to recharge our batteries. When we are walking in the country amongst nature, we are growing like the plants surrounding us. While we are "green" we are growing is an old saying. Let us learn from nature around us and marvel in awe at God's creations.

Why do animals exercise?

Animals in the wild need no doctors, no chiropractors and no physiotherapists. Why is that you might ask? Animals exercise all day. To survive, they walk, run and forage for their food. They don't sit on chairs or lounge suites. Animals are fit all of their life because of their way of their life.

Why should we exercise?

Let us learn a life lesson from animals to focus more time on exercise so we spend less time with doctors and other health professionals. While we are exercising, our fitness is growing and this helps us lead a longer and healthier life.

To create more energy

EXERCISE = ENERGY
MORE EXERCISE = MORE ENERGY
NO EXERCISE = NO ENERGY

To eliminate toxins

Drinking eight glasses of water each day will help clean out the toxins in our system and by exercising every day, such as walking, will help clean our blood, stomach and lymphatic system of toxins. Exercise helps keep us regular. If our bowels are emptied on a daily basis once or twice a day, this lessens the chances of disease in our body. Many diseases can start from constipation building up in the colon and that is why exercising every day helps clean out the colon. The lower the toxic load you have in your body the longer you will live. Toxins are the perfect breeding ground for bacteria to multiply in your body. The combination of alkaline food, sufficient water and daily exercise will make you clean on the inside, increasing your chances of a longer life.

To lose weight

A powerful motivation to exercise is to lose weight. We know we need to burn calories to lose weight. The hardest thing to do in our life is to face ourselves and ask questions. How did I put on so much weight? We need to let go of blame and try to get to the root cause of the problem. It is not easy to face ourselves. Transformation begins when we try to understand our self. What emotions do we need to change, do we need to let go of past experiences? At some point we may realize we can only change one day at a time. We need to look at changing our daily food habits. Instinctively, we know we need to eat more fruits and vegetables and less processed food. If exercise is a challenge for you, then you really need to be aware that you must change. Why not join a gym with like-minded people? Other people can give you the inspiration to lose weight. If you prefer individual training why not invest in a personal trainer. The feeling of losing weight and an increase in self-esteem and positive attitude could be the best dividends you ever receive from an investment in your health.

How to get fit

Fitness by association

What you surround yourself with you will become, eventually. Be friendly with people who talk about fitness and health and you will become like them. They will become like a magnet to you attracting thoughts and discussions about fitness and health. Thought precedes action, so getting excited about fitness will push you with more energy towards action. Ask yourself what is stopping you from exercising? Your enemies are procrastination and laziness to get fired up to make a jumping start. Those internal enemies can be defeated. Other people have the ability to get over these barriers, why not you? Think about some famous movie stars like Silvester Stallone or Angelina Jolie. They did not start out with a healthy, trim and athletic body. Somewhere in their life there was a spark that ignited their interest in exercise, fitness and health. As their health and fitness grew, their self-esteem was nourished and blossomed like a flower reaching for the sky. Your purpose in life may unfold as exercise and health gives your life new meaning. Everything starts inside of you, therefore, let other people inspire you so that the energy created by exercise will show on the outside in your glowing face and dynamic finely tuned body.

Motivation is the key to fitness

Inspired to live a long life? Remember the Hunza people who have many people living to 100 years old? They lead by example, walking every day to their orchards, possibly 10 to 20 km every day. Look out your window early in the morning or late in the evening and you will see singles, couples and families with the courage to walk. It could be one km but they are doing it, "who dares wins". You don't need to walk a long distance. What is stopping you from getting your shoes on and getting the blood pumping, one foot after another out on the pavement. I believe you can do it!

Walking surrounded by birds and trees is your new paradise to discover. When you take up the challenge to walk you will notice new frontiers, for example, amazing new exotic flowers and trees in your neighbour's garden. Count how many brightly coloured birds you observe as you walk. Where did they come from and where are their nests? As you walk around think about yourself as an adventurer blazing new trails in your neighbourhood. Captain Cook and Christopher Columbus were spirited adventures discovering new countries so why not be a spirited explorer uncovering unknown territory in your own suburb. Walk down new streets and open your eyes to the beauty of the smell of lavender from freshly planted flowers. Marvel at bees gathering pollen from brightly painted flowers and wonder how they make honey without a factory.

Walking opens up opportunities about perspective about what you see in the world outside your house. Early in the morning, dare to smile and say hello to a stranger while walking. Even a simple smile has the ability to transform a fellow walker's life. They may have challenges in their life and giving them a smile could lift their eyes from looking down at the mud to once again looking with awe at the sky and the stars above. I have planted the seed of motivation in you with words. It is now time for you to add some sunshine of awareness and the flow of water to the seed. Let your seed of exercise burst forth in action to begin the journey of walking.

Priority fitness defeats the TV

What is your priority today, more TV or more life energy? Energy is created by movement and fitness energizes your body from the inside. TV is a time trap. What you do with your time today creates your future. Now watching a certain amount of TV won't do you any harm. How much time do you spend watching TV? Spending 20 minutes a day exercising is depositing a longer time in your personal bank account of life on earth. Happiness is created by what we do and what we focus on. You can't get fresh air from a TV and you won't smell the perfume of flowers from watching either. Open the front door of your house into a new world with your walking shoes for traction. Fill your lungs with oxygen supplied by trees and as you walk focus on your heart pumping inside of you keeping you alive. Fill your senses with fragrant aromas from the abundant gardens surrounding your neighbours. Feel the sun tingle your skin adding vitamin D to strengthen your bones. As your walking pace quickens your flow of blood charges oxygen to every vital organ in your body. It is like recharging your mobile phone with a reserve of energy. You were given a healthy body at birth and what you do with it is up to you and your daily priorities. Ponder carefully to choose wisely what you do with your time. The important decisions we make about our body each day will make us or break us in the long term.

Swimming

Swimming is one of the aerobic exercises that can be fun, practiced by all age groups and even people with joint pain or arthritis or those recovering from a major disease such as a heart attack.

Swimming three times a week for at least an hour will give you dynamic energy and will:

- Strengthen your heart
- Help improve the circulation of your blood, especially if you have clogged arteries
- Over time, increase your lung capacity and help prevent asthma
- Potentially help cure conditions like asthma, for example, one of my friends in primary school Stephen was cured of asthma after swimming for a period of time
- Cool you down in the hotter seasons of the year and, during winter, if a heated pool is available where you live, it will help

warm and oxygenate your body, especially if it is too cold outside for walking

- Exercise your whole body, because swimming is a dynamic aerobic activity
- Increase the strength of your body without putting pressure on any particular muscle group
- Help ease joint problems, arthritis and osteoporosis (like hydrotherapy)
- Improve the flexibility of your body.

Exercise is one of the key habits of people who live to be 100 years old.

When are you going to get motivated to exercise?

Now? Or when you are in hospital suffering from a heart attack?

Tai Chi

History of Tai Chi

Tai Chi was developed in China in the 13th century reputedly by a monk called Chang San Feng.

The symbol of Tai Chi is a circle which shows the yin and the yang joined together. Yin is the male active energy and yang is the female passive energy. They are opposite of each other, i.e. positive and negative, light and day, good and bad.

Tai Chi is fantastic for young and old. Many years ago a friend of mine who had retired a couple of years earlier was showing signs of Alzheimer's disease. He started Tai Chi and after a short time his energy levels improved, his powers of concentration were enhanced, his focus became sharper and he developed a more positive outlook on life.

The benefits of Tai Chi

- Abundant energy
- More focused
- Sleep more deeply
- Less stress
- Increased flexibility
- More joy in your life
- Balance grows in your life
- Peace of mind
- Spiritual growth
- Keeps brain active
- Improves powers of concentration

My beautiful wife and I attended a three-day health seminar at Hopewood Health Retreat at Penrith near Sydney. During the retreat there was a Tai Chi demonstration at Hopewood by a man who had been practising Tai Chi for more than 15 years. When he asked the audience for a volunteer, a lady who had experienced severe pain in her hip stepped forward. The Tai Chi expert explained how he was about transfer "Chi" energy into her hip areas and then placed his hands on the painful areas. Within minutes the lady said her pain had reduced significantly. When are you going to experience the health benefits of Tai Chi?

Cycling

Cycling is a low cost aerobic exercise that gets the heart pumping more and helps improve the circulation of the blood. It is an Olympic sport that if you practice will help develop your stamina, endurance and strength and perhaps you could even set a goal to win a gold medal at the next Olympic games.

In Australia, many new housing estates have concrete cycling tracks clearly marked on the left side or on the normal walking path. You could also choose to cycle on the road at a time early in the morning or in the evening when there are not as many cars on the road. Start slowly and build up to 30 to 40 minute cycling sessions. I believe you can do it! Be daring until you find the type of exercise you are comfortable with.

Benefits of cycling

- Aerobic exercise
- Burns calories and helps weight loss
- Breathing more deeply helps improve your lung capacity
- Allows you to explore your local neighbourhood
- Great for building stamina and endurance
- Takes you away from the TV screen into the real world
- Causes you to sweat and opens the pores of your skin thus removing internal toxins.

ACT Action Creates Transformation

1. To discover if your fitness level is improving you need to start with a good look at how your body is now. This could be a scary thought for some. You need to be brave enough to face yourself in the mirror and start with the present moment. What you record you will reward. This means you need to keep a **fitness diary**. The reward in increasing fitness is more energy, more life, stronger self-esteem, more confidence, better feelings, a healthier heart, better circulation and a longer life. The question is, are you willing to pay the price in self-discipline?

2. In your fitness diary, record your weight. If you are overweight, you need to burn calories by daily exercise, that is, burning more calories by exercise than the calories of the food you are eating. Get motivated as this could be the turning point of your life, if you are ready to make a huge

change in your life. Record your weight in your fitness diary on a weekly basis.

3. Healthy heart, healthy life. Your goal is to lower your heart rate over a period of time. This means purchasing a digital blood pressure machine that measures resting heart rate. You can get one in Australia for about $80 to $100. This is an investment in your future health. Record your resting heart rate in your fitness diary on a weekly basis.

4. Your fitness diary is an important tool to keep you on track with a written record of your achievements.

Examples of entries in a fitness diary:

SEPTEMBER

5 Monday

> 12.00 am – 12.30 pm: Walking
> 8.00 pm – 8.30 pm: Stretching, Tai Chi, yoga, 2 kg bar bell lifting

6 Tuesday

> 12.00 am – 12.30 pm: Walking
> 8.00 pm – 8.30 pm: Stretching, Tai Chi, yoga, 2 kg bar bell lifting

7 Wednesday

> 12.00 am – 12.30 pm: Walking
> 8.00 pm – 8.30 pm: Stretching, Tai Chi, yoga, 2 kg bar bell lifting

8 Thursday

> 12.00 am – 12.30 am: Walking

9 Friday

> 6.30 pm – 7.00 pm: Walking to shops

10 Saturday

> 7.00 am – 8.00 am: Walking around your neighbourhood
> 8.00 pm – 8.30 pm: Stretching, Tai Chi, yoga, 2 kg bar bell lifting

11 Sunday

> 7.00 am – 8.00 am: Walking around neighbourhood
> 7.30 pm: Record blood pressure and resting heart rate and your weight (this is part of the truth serum of facing yourself in the mirror)
> 8.00 pm – 8.30 pm Tai Chi Yoga

Remember: what is recorded gets done and you can see your actual achievements.

5. If motivating yourself is a problem, start walking with your wife or husband and you will inspire each other. The couple who exercise together stays together.
6. A gym is a great place to see and meet other people who can inspire you to start a fitness program. Some people get more motivated when they see other people on a similar journey.
7. Our life is an adventure when we try new experiences. You never know how your energy levels and overall health can be transformed by daring to try a new exercise:

   - Yoga
   - Tai Chi
   - Swimming
   - Dancing
   - Lifting weights

- Golf
- Tennis
- Basketball
- Walking.

Who dares wins for a longer, disease-free life.

There are two voices inside of you:
The voice of the angel
And the voice of the beast.
Whichever you feed the most
Wins!

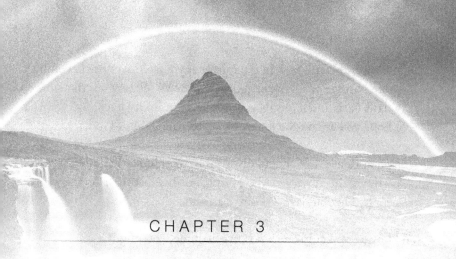

CHAPTER 3

ATTITUDE

In the journey to live to be 100 years old, mind body and spirit work together. One thing in common in cultures with greater longevity like the Hunza people and the Okinawa people is they have very positive attitudes, they are happy people and laugh a lot.

Your attitude is the seed of what you have grown inside of you. Your attitude is either positive or negative. If your focus is mostly fear, doubt, revenge, criticism, lack, gossip, jealousy, hate, anger and what is wrong with the world, then people could say you have a negative attitude. If your focus is courage, hope, faith, forgiveness, appreciation, love and self-control, then people could say you have a positive attitude.

We are not perfect so we have a mixture of positive and negative attitudes inside of us. We have two voices inside of us, the voice leading to the light, e.g. faith, hope and love and the voice leading us into the darkness, e.g. doubt, fear and hate.

Whichever you feed the most will dominate your life. Wisely choose your thoughts, as moment by moment, day by day they are creating your future. We are on a journey to the light or on a journey to the darkness. Have a look in the mirror at yourself. Are you becoming a more positive or a more negative person? We choose our thoughts on a daily basis and it is only you who has the ability to change yourself. I hope you are on the journey towards the light of God.

When Renee Taylor actually lived in the Hunza Valley for a period of time, she observed the strong positive attitude of the Hunza people. Do you have a positive attitude?

How do you cultivate a positive attitude, you might ask?

A positive attitude means you have

- Hope
- Faith
- Love
- Peace of mind
- Harmony
- Compassion
- A sharing attitude
- Persistence
- Tolerance
- Happiness
- A generous attitude
- Self-control
- A friendly nature
- Forgiveness
- Courage
- Wisdom.

Hope

Building a house means adding one brick at a time. Likewise, we build a positive mental attitude one thought at a time.

Hope is looking forward to a better life. As we get older we are either getting better or bitter. I hope you choose to get better.

You are building hope with each thought you think. If a doubting thought enters your mind, gently replace the thought with the hope that your life is improving: I hope my life is improving, I have hope that my life is improving. Hope is a higher quality thought for you and your future.

What you build inside of you will show up on the outside of your life eventually. Therefore, intentionally build a positive attitude inside of you.

Go to the beach and watch the waves persistently wearing away the rocks of doubt. We are hoping to be healthy and live to be 100 years old. This means we are starting to cultivate more positive thoughts and transforming into the action of eating more alkaline forming foods and less acidic forming foods. When we eat more alkaline forming food, e.g. vegetables, greens, fruits and nuts which contain abundant vitamins, minerals and fibre, we are building a fortress of young healthy and energetic cells inside our bodies and slowly we will have more energy and vitality on the outside and other people will notice this new vitality.

In the journey of how to live to be 100 years old, the number one most powerful positive emotion is love and most cultures with greater longevity like the Hunza people are full of love and display very little hate. Could it be that love can conquer crime? There is very little crime in most longevity cultures and they are mostly full of married people with very few divorced people.

Could John Lennon's song 'All You Need is Love' be the answer to many of life's challenges?

Love

"There are three things that last forever faith, hope and love. But the greatest of all is love." – 1 Corinthians 13:13

What is love?

The source of love is God so if you have love inside you then you have God inside you. We can only give another person what is inside of us. We can seek love in the outside world only to discover that we need to love ourselves first. Loving yourself means you take care of your mind, body and spirit. When we can take care of ourselves, we can take care of our loved ones.

Remember, loving ourselves is not selfish love, as we can only give to others what we already have inside of us. When there is only love inside you, others will sense the aroma of peace, love and harmony in your spirit. Love attracts love from the universe surrounding us and when there is hate inside you, then you will attract hate from the universe like a magnet.

What do you want to attract from the universe surrounding you, LOVE or HATE?

Cultivate thoughts and emotions of love and your world will slowly be filled with loving people. Whereas, if you cultivate bitter thoughts of hate and resentment and your world will slowly be filled with hateful and resentful people. Choose wisely your thoughts and emotions, because, as your thoughts and emotions change so does the world around you change.

Marriage rainbow

A good marriage must be created
In the art of marriage the little things, are the big things.
It is never being too old to hold hands

It is remembering to say "I LOVE YOU" at least once a day
It is never going to sleep angry
It is a mutual sense of values and common objectives
It is speaking words of appreciation and showing gratitude in thoughtful ways
It is the capacity to forgive and forget
It is finding room for the things of the spirit
It is not only marrying the right partner
It is being the right partner.

Practical demonstrations of love

Love is …

- Buying your wife some healthy dark chocolate and a bottle of romantic red wine and having a candlelight dinner together
- Helping your partner with domestic work
- Being the first to say sorry in a disagreement
- Looking at the other person's point of view
- Buying small gifts for your loving partner
- Sharing in looking after the children
- Exercising together
- Hugging each other more often
- Kissing each other more often
- Making love not war
- Listening to each other without judging what is said
- Being kind to each other
- Forgiving the partner first because we are all human
- Caring for each with signs of affection
- Helping each other during the many challenges of life
- Giving compassion to each other during difficult times
- Going on a date with each other every week even if you have been married for a very long time.

Remember your world changes when you change.

RECIPE FOR LOVE

Ingredients

1 cup of Romance
1 pinch of Humour
2 tsp of Joy
1 lb of Compatibility
3 tb of Trust
1 cup of Respect
½ lb of Sharing
1 zest of Tenderness
¾ cup of Patience

Peace of Mind

People who live to be 100 years old besides loving each other, have another thing in common, they have cultivated having more peace of mind in regard to themselves their family and their local community. When you are at peace with yourself then you will be at peace with your partner, your neighbour and the universe. When you at war with yourself, you will be at war with your partner, your neighbour and the universe. We attract from the universe only what is inside of us. Listen to that small inner voice inside of us and let us practice cultivating a spirit of peace of mind.

Peace is like deep water; it is calm on the surface and like deep water it sees deeply into the treasures of life inside us. Peace is the absence of stress; when we find peace we find the presence of God.

Trees grow in silence and peace. There is peace in the silence of the planets orbiting the sun. God created the planets and the sun; there is divine order in the universe. Cultivate peace of mind and divine order will slowly grow like a seed in your life.

Peace is the absence of war. The sun sends rays of light 93 million miles away in silence and in peace. The more silence you have and the more peace of mind you cultivate, the more light you are giving to the people around you. Thinking peaceful thoughts attracts peace and thinking war-like thoughts attracts war, slowly but surely over a period of time.

The birds of the air have peace of mind as they trust in God every day to provide food, water and shelter. They do not work, they pay no rent and have no mortgage yet they have peace of mind. What can we learn from the birds that sing with happiness every day at the crack of dawn?

The more we cultivate peace of mind, each and every day, the healthier we become and the longer our life will be. Choose your thoughts wisely. When we choose peaceful thoughts, we attract a happy and joyful life. What are you attracting in your life right now?

Faith

Cultures with greater longevity have another thing in common, they have faith in themselves and they also have faith that there is a God, no matter what particular religion they may follow. God is the one who controls the universe, who else can maintain control of the universe with all its galaxies, stars and planets?

When we have faith in God, faith in ourselves and faith in the unfolding of our particular journey in life, we have the awareness that comes from dwelling in the light. What is your main focus, faith and trust in God and the universe, or doubt and cynicism and living in darkness and despair?

Doubting thoughts create barriers in our life and we tend to attract more problems and difficulties. When we complain more and more, the universe sends us more things to complain about.

When we appreciate and have gratitude, more and more in our life, the universe gives us more things to be grateful for, slowly but surely. Ralph Waldo Emerson calls this the Law of Compensation.

If we want a long and disease-free life, we need to be responsible for our actions, that are in fact our habits, that lead us to a longer healthy life. There is no point blaming others for our sickness, negative thought patterns, or lack of commitment to changing our life. All that happens in our life flows from our thoughts, feelings and attitudes. Longevity is about balancing our mind, body and spirit and especially our thoughts and feelings. Faith, hope and love are the strongest positive emotions to cultivate. Having faith builds our belief that we are building a healthy body by exercise, a healthy mind by choosing our thoughts wisely and building our spirit by loving everybody and accepting everybody the way they are without judging them. Respect everybody and they will respect you.

Our body is like a temple. When we grow faith in us, slowly but surely, we create dynamic energy inside us. Then, what we fill the temple of our body with begins to change. We begin to change our eating habits, thought habits, and exercise habits. Consequently, the universe gives us a healthy disease-free body, longer life and abundant energy.

MORE ENERGY AND MORE FAITH = A LONGER AND PAIN FREE LIFE

Growing a positive attitude

Growing a positive attitude inside of us will help shield us from fear, worry and anxiety.

> Sorrow looks back
> Worry looks around
> Faith looks up
>
> *Anonymous*

Positive mind

When you choose more positive thoughts over negative thoughts, eventually, you will develop a positive mind. Yes, this takes time but just like a small seed can grow into a mighty tree, you can do it when you change your habits of thought over time. I can do it so you can as well. The world looks very different with your positive glasses on and you tend to look for the rainbow after the storms of life rather than focusing on the lightning and thunder. Your focus becomes your life. Focus on living a long healthy disease-free life and you are already on the path to achieving a positive mind.

You feed your body with nourishing food to provide your body with energy, but do you feed your mind with a positive or negative thought diet?

Just like plants need sunshine and water to flourish, we need to be careful what we feed our mind. Is this a stream of negative thoughts, e.g. doubt, complaints, gossip, and criticism of others? These types of thoughts slowly but surely attract circumstances of life that will give us more problems, lack of energy, depression and a sick body.

In contrast, when we feed our mind on a diet of faith, gratitude, appreciation, love, hope and courage, the universe will slowly attract the circumstances of life that reflect back to us our thoughts like a mirror.

In the evening news, we see violence, tragedy, sickness, war, accidents and basically, what is wrong with the world. After a daily diet of this news, it is almost as if we expect to see these things in our daily life.

What would happen if, instead of watching the stories on TV about what is wrong with the world, we communicated with our family and shared the stories of our day? Listening to and sharing stories with our loved ones builds trust, sharing, hope, love, faith and peace of mind at our dinner table. By doing this, we are building up and appreciating each other, having a laugh with each other and sharing problems that can be solved by others with more experience and wisdom.

God controls the universe and it is your
attitude that controls your life.
The universe only changes when we change.
Are you ready to change?

Source *Unknown*

Laughter

A sense of humour is an attitude that also improves our chances of achieving longevity.

To commemorate her birthday, Julie Andrews once made a special appearance at the Manhattan City Music Hall. One of the musical numbers she performed was 'My Favourite Things' from the much loved movie 'The Sound of Music'. Here are the lyrics with a twist:

Botox and nose drops and needles for knitting. Walkers and handrails and new dental fittings. Bundles of magazines tied up in string. These are a few of my favourite things. Cadillacs and cataracts, and hearing aids and glasses. Polident and Fixodent and false teeth in glasses. Pacemakers, golf carts and porches with swings, these are a few of my favourite things. When the pipes leak, when the bones creak, when the knees go bad. I simply remember my favourite things and then I don't feel so bad.

The old saying is true: "Laughter is the best medicine!"

ACT   Action Creates Transformation

1. Gratitude. For three months change your attitude and try to become more positive and see if your world changes. On waking in the morning, spend the first five minutes thanking God for your blessings.

    For example:

    *   Thank you for the gift of life
    *   Thank you for my abundant health
    *   Thank you for love flowing into my life
    *   Thank you for peace of mind
    *   Thank you for food, water and shelter

- Thank you for giving me a loving wife
- Thank you for my job
- Thank you for a safe trip to work in my car
- Thank you for abundance flowing into my life

2. Eat a healthy breakfast to give yourself more energy in your day.

   Alkaline Breakfast + Positive Attitude = More Energy in Your Day

3. Spend more time appreciating the people in your life and less time criticizing people.

   Starting today, try this for the next three months. Remember, you are making a change in your life so be persistent and the more you appreciate other people, the more you will be appreciated, whereas, the more you criticize other people, the more you will be criticized.

4. This week, develop an attitude of walking for 30 minutes for three times over the next seven days. You will benefit by an increase in energy and your stress levels will decrease.

   Remember: WHO DARES WINS – motto of SAS Commandos.

5. Create fun activities in your life with your partner and friends.

   Make a date with your partner for a romantic meal and remember when you fell in love with your partner. Have a coffee with a close friend this week. Spend more time with your children this week.

6. Have a drive in the country and be inspired by the mountains or the beach and walk in a forest and be inspired by mother nature. Take time to smell the roses.

7. Take time to laugh and have fun. Being around children and their infectious laughter will certainly put a smile on your face.

When the student is ready
The teacher will appear.

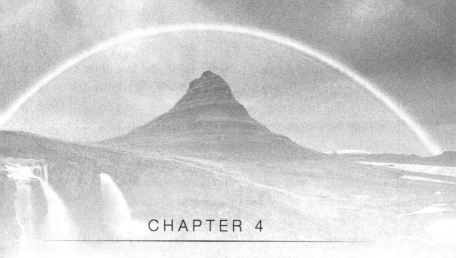

LIFE-LONG LEARNING

In the journey to live to be 100 years old, we need to be like a young evergreen tree with bright green leaves. While you are green you are growing in wisdom, knowledge and understanding. Also, your brain cells will have increased activity levels that keep your brain alive and lessen chance of you acquiring the diseases of age like Alzheimer's disease.

The benefits of life-long learning

Especially if you are in your senior years, you would have spent a great deal of time, money and energy focusing on paying bills and keeping up with the rent or mortgage payments. Now is the time to get back on the learning curve and embrace life-long learning. Life becomes exciting again when we study a new skill, learn a new language, learn how to play a musical instrument and set some learning goals to expand our life and our future. When you are learning new skills, your inner world starts to expand again as you are meeting new people, learning from them and sharing our new skills and experiences with your friends and the community of people with whom you circulate.

This helps us to understand change is inevitable and we need to let go of fear for the future and replace it with an optimistic outlook that our life is getting better because we are getting better by building our character and actively pursuing new skills which expand our world.

It is not wise to rest on our laurels and think we know everything just because we might be in our senior years. Even the famous philosopher Socrates said, there is always something new to learn. So if you are 20, 30, 40, 50, 60, 70, 80, 90 or even a 100, you can learn new things every single day.

As we get into our senior years, we either get cynical about life and complain all the time or become wiser and appreciate life with gratitude. We can also give back to the community by sharing what we have learnt. It is important to share our time, treasure and talent. Emerson said, "The more you give to others, the more the universe will give back to you, especially if you don't expect something back in return." Slowly, we are learning the lessons of life that will help lead us to live to be 100 years old.

Learning in our early life

Correct breathing technique

What is the first lesson of life you learnt after emerging from your mother's womb? You learnt how to breathe. Babies breathe using their diaphragm and there is wisdom in this method of breathing as it allows the maximum amount of oxygen into our lungs and then into our bloodstream helping to increase the alkaline nature of our blood. Later in life, you will learn that people who study martial arts and yoga know the impact and importance of diaphragm breathing for the whole body.

Learning about love

Your life-long journey of adventure in the world begins when you move from the darkness of the womb to the bright lights surrounding you in the hospital delivery room; your five senses are challenged by new sounds and smells. You feel the love flowing from your mother's first hug and long embrace. Nourishment flows from your mother's breast as you taste your first meal in the world outside of your mother's womb.

Your first meal is alkaline

Amazingly, breast milk is alkaline and in this, God gives us a clue as to what type of food will help us live a long, healthy and happy life. Breast milk will be your only food for the next 12 months at least. God knows in his wisdom what our body needs.

Lesson of persistence and determination

A big challenge is awaiting you over the next 12 months as you first learn to crawl and eventually you learn to stand up and walk on your own two feet with the encouragement of your mum and dad. In your life-long learning journey you are now learning an important lesson that you will need all of your life. You struggle to stand up on your own, you fall down but with courage you try again, you try to stand up and you fall again.

Lesson of no fear

Hopefully you can see the important lesson: NEVER, NEVER GIVE UP. At this young age you are fearless and don't recognize dangers that surround you. At home you climb the lounge suite and jump on to the floor not knowing the hurt that it may cause your body. Your first teachers are your mum and dad and they will teach you all they know.

Learning to communicate

The next challenge is to begin communicating with your mum and dad. Your parents encourage you to speak. Your mum and dad are radiant with joy and happiness as you utter your first words such as "mum mum". As time goes by, more communication skills are added including writing and drawing which are important additions to your life.

You are on a steep learning curve as you rapidly accumulate a vocabulary of words to allow you to more fully connect with your mum and dad, as well as the world around you. Self-control is also learnt as you slowly master the workings of the human body.

Learning independence

Independence is learnt as you finally can feed yourself, put on your own clothes and master self-discipline, an important lesson for your future. You learn to let go of your mum and dad as you attend primary school and later high school. Realisation slowly dawns on you of the importance of education for a successful future.

Understand yourself first then other people

You start to look in the mirror to discover what is inside of your spirit and to learn your strengths and weaknesses in relation to capturing your first job. Many important life lessons are learnt in dealing with the opposite sex and working as a team with other people. Intuition is guiding you to your future job, and realizing that your mum and dad have wisdom that comes with age, you learning to stand on your own two feet to face the world.

What does TEAM stand for?

- Together
- Everybody

- Achieves
- More

Preparing for a job

Formal life-long learning begins.

We leave high school and realize we have only just begun to start learning. Depending on our purpose and direction in life, we may begin an apprenticeship and become a tradesman in the future or perhaps study at university or TAFE college and eventually become a professional such as

- an accountant
- a builder
- a carpenter
- a doctor
- a hairdresser
- a teacher
- an IT professional
- a plumber
- a sales person
- a cook
- a manager
- receptionist.

We might even start our own business if we have that entrepreneurial spirit. Deep inside of us there is the knowledge of what we will become so we need to dig deep for the "GOLD" inside of us whispering our future job. After our formal studies, we begin our first job and learn skills from others in the workforce. We learn "people skills", computer skills, teamwork and as we make mistakes, we learn our own lessons of life.

The workplace is undergoing great changes: manufacturing jobs are disappearing as we are importing more and making things less in our own country, and as automation takes over, many jobs are automated, e.g. the cashier at the supermarket is replaced by a machine. In the car industry, manual labour is being replaced by welding robots, and retail shops are disappearing and going on the internet.

When the workplace changes we need to change

At the same time, opportunities are growing as we realize we can adapt and change and learn new skills. The era of one job for life in many industries is vanishing. What opportunities are there, you might ask?

Many people now are employed in service industries, e.g. teachers, cleaners, chefs, waiters, kitchen hands, IT roles, and trades such as plumbers, electricians and hairdressers.

Many people start their own business, e.g. consultants, coffee shops, café owners, cleaners, web site designers and boot camp trainers.

Life-long learning means learning new skills all of the time.

Remember, there is a lot of competition in the workplace for the available jobs. If you are not learning new skills, your fellow job seekers are so WHY AREN'T YOU?

My own working life has seen some dramatic changes:

1. Instrument fitter
2. Quality control inspector
3. Metallurgist
4. Technical officer in the aircraft industry
5. Tutoring high school students

6. Business trainer
7. Author

WHEN WE CHANGE, THE WORLD APPEARS TO CHANGE

Personalities

Life-long learning is also about learning about people and relationships, especially the people we love: our marriage partner, children, friends and family. There are four main personality types that can help you to understand yourself and other people.

1. Choleric

The born leader, the dominant personality, the decision maker, and strong willed.

"My way or the highway" is a common phrase used by the choleric personality.

E.g. Winston Churchill and Margaret Thatcher.

2. Sanguine

Let's have fun, loves to talk, good sense of humour, storyteller, and emotional.

"I will tell you a story" is a common phrase used by the sanguine personality.

E.g. Lucille Ball and Chevy Chase.

3. Phlegmatic

Calm, cool and collected, peaceful, loves to listen, and balanced.

"Let us watch and see what happens" is a common phrase used by the phlegmatic personality.

E.g. Ronald Regan and Gerald Ford (both former US presidents).

4. Melancholy

Analytical, deep, genius, serious, and thinkers.

"If it's worth doing, it's worth doing right" is a common phrase used by the melancholy personality.

E.g. Michelangelo and Picasso.

LIVING WATER

*Jesus said to the woman at the well,
"I will give them living water
gushing within..."
John 4: 13-15*

ACT   Action Creates Transformation

1. Spend one day in quiet and silence. This might not be something you normally do, however, if you do, you are opening yourself up to the small voice within you that knows your future purpose and direction for your life.

2. After examining your life, make a decision. Perhaps, you might decide your present job has no future and you need to study to be a chef, a beautician, a small business owner, to run a market stall, be a fitness trainer, a handyman, a website designer, an artist, a renovator, a nail technician, a massage therapist, a kitchen hand or a barista. Make a written goal and outline the steps as a road map to achieve your goal with a timeline to achieve your goal. For example,

   a. GOAL: I will be a chef by ___/___/_____ (set a specific date).

   b. Step 1: Enrol at TAFE or university in a course for the specific trade or profession you are aiming for.

   c. Step 2: Make sacrifices by studying three nights per week for this course.

   d. Step 3: Find a mentor – somebody who has already achieved the job and who you admire. E.g. read their books about how they got started and how they overcame their challenges to finally succeed at their job.

   e. Step 4: Be persistent and never give up on your dream job and remember that one step beyond your greatest challenge is your greatest success.

   f. Step 5: First thing in the morning, read out aloud your written goal three times and last thing at night before you go to bed, read your goal again three times. Imagine in your mind that you have already achieved your goal. When you imagine your goal in your mind, you will start to see opportunities around you that lead towards you achieving your goal. Never give up on your goal.

3. Examine your strengths and weaknesses in your current job. If you feel that this is the job that you love, take note of your weaknesses and take action to improve them. Most people

love to look at other people weaknesses but refuse to look at their own weaknesses. Improving your weaknesses at work is the quickest way for you to be successful in the long term. Self-improvement is the best investment you will ever make in your life.

4. When you discover the job you love you will be happier, healthier, have more energy and live a longer life.

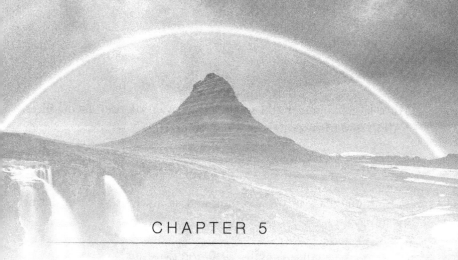

CHAPTER 5

DRINK PURE WATER

What is the miracle of drinking pure water?

The Romanian Nobel Prize winner in fluid dynamics, Dr Henri Coanda, spent over 50 years studying the water from the Hunza Valley to try to discover its miraculous components.

What Dr Coanda did discover was that the water was alkaline with a high pH and a high colloidal mineral content (rich mineral content). These same water properties can be found in other unpolluted areas around the world, e.g. near Azerbaijan (close to Russia) and in the Andes Mountains (South America). Both the Azerbaijan people and the Vilcabamba people (of the Andes) are known for their longevity and the unusual numbers of 100-year-old plus people in their communities.

Recipe for alkaline water

One litre carbon filtered water (use tap water if filtered water is not available)
One teaspoon Himalayan salt (alkalinity ~pH 9)
One sliced lemon (please don't squeeze the lemon slices)

Garry Gordon

Procedure

In a large container add water, Himalayan salt and lemon slices. Allow to settle overnight at room temperature.

Action

Drink one glass in the morning and as much as you can during your day.

Take up the challenge to live to be 100 years old.

Benefits of pure water

- Abundant ENERGY
- Vitality
- Fullness of life
- More oxygen in your blood
- Reduce bone and joint pain
- Your kidneys will last longer
- Lowers risk of Alzheimer's disease and dementia
- Reduce acidity in your body
- Reduce risk of disease

There are so many benefits to drinking pure water.

How much pure water did you drink today?

Drink pure water

The two best choices in drinking pure water to achieve a lifespan of 100 years old are:

1. Drink pure filtered water at least 1.5 litres per day. Don't think about it but actually START DOING IT NOW!

2. Drink ALKALINE WATER like the Hunza people do. It is not what you read that changes your life it is what you DO that counts.

In Australia, the closest you can get to drinking pure water is filtering your water with a carbon filter to remove impurities like chlorine, lead and other heavy metals.

I personally know two people who have been hospitalized because of drinking tap water. Tests in hospital showed they had giardia bacteria and they were both sick for a long period of time before they recovered.

How pure is the water you drink every day?

- Our body is about 70% water it needs your awareness to supply it with the best and most pure water every day to maintain abundant health and reduce the risk of a major sickness like kidney disease, cancer or heart attack.
- Your blood is about 90% water.
- Your brain is about 85% water and lack of water can lead to Alzheimer's disease.

The positive benefits of drinking pure water

1. You will have more energy and vitality. You will feel like there is an internal waterfall flowing within you.
2. Improved kidney function and less chance of kidney disease and kidney stones. Your kidneys filter your blood and your blood is about 90% water. If you want your kidneys to last a lifetime, drink more pure water and live to be 100 years old.
3. Improved weight loss because in order to lose weight, the fat can only exit your body by urine, excreta and through the pores of your skin. Drinking pure water vastly increases the process of losing weight through urination and excreta. Let us be practical, how else will the fat leave your body?

4. Reduced risk of dying from cancer. Cancer loves an acidic bloodstream and the stomach and colon can be the beginning of most diseases including cancer. When the intestines are blocked with faeces through constipation, cancer and other diseases can start to grow because of the build-up of bacteria and toxins. Pure water allows the intestines to transport the waste out of the body much more easily, especially if you eat enough fibre in your daily intake of food as well.

5. Models with glowing skin drink plenty of water as this naturally hydrates the skin and helps the skin to be more elastic. When you look better on the outside, your self-esteem will also improve.

6. Many people who suffer headaches are dehydrated. Think about this: your brain is about 85% water and if you are not drinking enough pure water, it is like your brain is shrinking due to lack of water. This is why one of the causes of headache is lack of water.

7. At work, sometimes your concentration and focus starts to decline but drinking more pure water can start to turn this around. Sometimes this decline in concentration can also be due to low blood sugar, especially around 10 am and 2.30 pm. Drinking more pure water will help you to focus more on the present moment.

8. Cramps and joint problems can result from insufficient pure water. Cramps can also be due to not enough magnesium in your daily food.

9. Exercise will benefit you more when more pure water is consumed because you sweat it out of your body and it needs replacing to continue to fuel your body.

10. Digestion is greatly improved with more pure water in your body. Think about this: all food is digested in your body and how does digestion get better? You need water and fibre to lubricate your intestines to smoothly remove the waste material from your body.

Yendel'ora
Place of Peace

As you sit here, quietly reflect on the Aboriginal people for whom this was a place of peace. Each generation gathered here from all over South Eastern Australia to resolve conflicts, to define the law and to foster peace between people.

Finding my own peace close to the gushing water of Yendel'ora.

ACT   Action Creates Transformation

1. Start to slowly to reduce drinking carbonated soft drinks from your daily routine and replace them with filtered water. If you are wondering why, then I suggest you buy some pH papers and see how acidic your carbonated soft drinks are really. The more acidic fluids you drink, the greater the chances of disease. Cancer thrives in an acidic bloodstream and one of the causes of osteoporosis is the body taking calcium (alkaline mineral) from your bones to increase the alkalinity of your bloodstream.

2. Drink green tea as green tea has many health benefits such as high antioxidant levels and is mostly water.

3. Watermelon is one of the most alkaline forming fruits you can eat and is mostly water.

4. Moderation in all things is a wise saying so if you drink too much coffee, slowly replace it with more healthy alternatives such as coconut water.

Enzymes add dynamic energy
to your body and a longer life

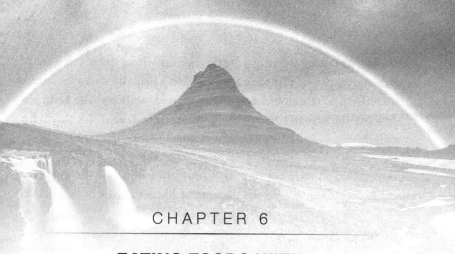

CHAPTER 6

EATING FOODS WITH ABUNDANT ENZYMES

One of the most important health pioneers who I admire the most is Ann Wigmore as she unfolded the healing secrets of wheat grass.

What is wheatgrass?

If you take an ordinary grain of wheat used to make bread and you plant it in the soil and nourish it with water and let the sun shine on the young plant, when the sprout emerges from the soil let it grow about 6 inches high (it will look like a long blade of grass) then cut the wheat just above the soil and you have WHEAT GRASS.

When you have many six inch long wheat grasses, you juice the wheat grass to get about 30 ml of wheatgrass juice. This juice "Elixir of the Gods" contains some of the most potent healing properties of any liquid on planet Earth.

Wheat grass juice contains abundant enzymes and has amazing healing properties. Many years ago my wife was diagnosed with lupus which, to the best of my knowledge, is just about incurable.

We began taking 30 ml of freshly juiced wheat grass juice twice daily over a period of time and with God's help my wife was cured. Something to remember: just like any good medicine, the taste is a bit sour. The way to balance this sourness is to take it together with something sweet like a piece of watermelon or similar fruit.

Remember, you are consuming wheat grass juice for the enzymes and to be healed, not for the sweet taste like lemonade or soft drink.

What are enzymes?

Enzymes could be one of "natures secrets" to living a long pain-free life. Enzymes are the "life force" that keeps us alive. Enzymes are the building blocks that work day and night inside your body to help all of the chemical processes, e.g. digestion in your stomach, many liver enzymes that help filter the poisons from your blood and co enzyme 10 that your heart needs to stop you from having a heart attack.

Cooking food kills enzymes that are naturally found in the raw food. Raw good, therefore, contains the maximum amount of enzymes. The more raw food you eat the longer you will live. Think about it like this: raw food is still alive, e.g. a raw carrot is still alive, whereas, a cooked piece of meat is dead.

When you eat more foods that are alive you will stay alive longer, whereas, when you eat more foods that are dead you will die sooner. Note that humans are the only species on the planet who cook their food.

Cows, sheep, kangaroos, deer, lions and tigers all eat raw food. Lions don't eat KFC or roast their meals on the fire before eating it do they? In the wild, are their hundreds and thousands of sick animals? No, animals in the wild don't get sick very often. Why is this, is it because they only eat raw foods? How many animal hospitals are there in the wild? I am not talking about veterinary hospitals for domestic cats and dogs that are fed cooked food, but in the wild. When animals get sick in the wild what do they do? Some of them eat certain plants and herbs naturally found in the wild and they usually get healed. Let us humans have a close look at what foods contain abundant enzymes.

Some of the most important foods containing enzymes

- All sprouts, e.g. mung bean sprouts, wheat grass sprouts
- Wheat grass juice
- Yogurt, especially natural yogurt – Hunza people eat yogurt & kefir which is popular in some countries in Europe it contains more good bacteria than yogurt.
- Fermented cabbage, e.g. sauerkraut and kimchi
- Most raw foods
- Barley grass and juice.

Some of the most important enzymes

- Co enzyme 10. Much research has shown that when this enzyme is low in the body it can trigger a heart attack. As we get older our reserves of this enzyme decline rapidly.
- Liver enzymes, e.g. cytochrome.

Enzymes decline with age

As we get older, our bodies produce fewer enzymes. We were born with a certain amount of enzymes and just like a bank account, we can add enzymes by eating enzyme rich food, e.g. uncooked food, bean sprouts, and yogurt.

The more enzymes in your body the longer your life.

Are you eating enzyme rich food?

The pancreas gives digestive enzymes

The pancreas gives enzymes to the small intestine to help with digestion of food. The stomach uses a lot of energy and enzymes when food is broken down into minerals, fibre, protein and vitamins. Your enzyme bank account gets used up "spent" when food is digested and processed by your body. It is only you who can add enzymes into your body by choosing enzyme rich food.

Enzyme bank account

When you "spend" all of the enzymes in your body, e.g. by overeating as your body uses a massive amount of enzymes to digest the food you eat, then your enzyme bank account is bankrupt of enzymes. It has no credit card of enzymes to borrow more for the digestion of more food. Low enzymes could result in your early death. A wise choice is to eat more enzyme rich food, e.g. raw juices such as carrot and wheatgrass, and yogurt. The Hunza people eat an abundance of enzyme rich food.

RAW FOODS=ENZYMES=MORE
ENERGY AND LONGER LIFE

COOKED FOODS=NO ENZYMES=LESS
ENERGY AND SHORTER LIFE

Cooked food versus raw food

Cooking food kills enzymes and eating more raw food, e.g. salad and fruit adds an abundance of enzymes to your body. Overeating uses up your digestive enzymes, whereas, eating raw food reduces the need for digestive enzymes and, therefore, your enzymes are preserved because salads and fruit are easily digested while meat takes a long time to be digested.

The Pottenger cat experiment

Many famous health food books have mentioned the Pottenger cat experiment and for good reasons, e.g. *Raw Energy* by Leslie and Susannah Kenton. In the experiment, over 900 cats were split into two groups, the first group was fed cooked meat and pasteurized milk while the second group was fed raw meat and unpasteurized milk. This experiment lasted 10 years, over four generations of cats.

- **Cooked food.** The cats fed cooked food developed most of the major degenerative diseases found in humans, e.g. arthritis. In each new generation, the disease severity increased significantly and in the third generation the cats that ate cooked foods did not have kittens.
- **Raw food.** The cats fed raw foods produced disease-free healthy kittens for four generations. For more information refer to the Price-Pottenger Nutrition Foundation, La Mesa, California, USA.

This is one of the most astonishing examples of the amazing effects of raw food and the enzymes they contain, in comparison with cooked food.

Foods to consider adding to your diet

Sprouted seeds

Seeds are placed in a container, water is added to cover the seeds and the water is changed two or three times a day. After about four days, a sprout emerges from the seed. This dynamic sprout is full of enzymes that helps the body in digestion and heals the body of sickness. Please read Anne Wigmore's book, *The Hippocrates Diet and Health Program*. If you prefer to buy your sprouts from the supermarket, they are very economic to buy if you are on a budget.

Hunza people love sprouts

Traditionally, on a daily basis the Hunza people love to eat freshly sprouted seeds and this could be one of the reasons so many Hunza people live to be over 100 years old. When the seed actually germinates there is an explosive increase in vitamin B, vitamin E and vitamin C levels. Sprouts are also full of one of the most potent killers of cancer cells, nitriloside. Other foods rich in nitrilosides are dried apricots and apricot seeds which are found inside the hard apricot kernel.

Papaya and your stomach

Papaya (or paw paw) is a tropical fruit which tastes amazing and contains the enzyme papain. This enzyme helps people with digestive problems. Papain is very similar to an enzyme called pepsin which helps digest one of the most difficult things for the stomach to digest, that is, protein. Papain has an astonishing ability to absorb and help the body process protein-rich food such as meat.

Pineapple and your joints

Pineapple contains the enzyme bromelain which helps reduce or eliminate inflammation in the joints, particularly for those suffering from arthritis. Eating a couple of slices of fresh pineapple works much better than pineapple from a can.

Coenzyme Q10 and your heart

Coenzyme 10 is a powerful antioxidant first isolated in 1957 by Dr Frederick Crane from the mitochondria inside a beef heart. Professor Yamamura from Japan was the first to use the compound coenzyme 10 in the treatment of congestive heart failure, according to the excellent book *Coenzyme Q10 The Wonder Nutrient*. In this highly recommended book, it says that the reason behind many chronic diseases is the absence of coenzyme 10 in the body, particularly as we get older. A friend of mine who loved to work in the garden had a heart attack, but after the heart attack he could not lift a spade in the garden. He began taking a coenzyme 10 supplement and within a week he had the energy to again work in the garden he loved.

Yogurt and good bacteria in your stomach

Yogurt contains the good bacteria acidophilus and bifidus which have a dramatic effect on your digestion in your upper and lower intestines. People who have had digestive problems for years often experience a transformation in a short period of time after eating natural yogurt. Try to use natural yogurt without added fruit. If after a one or two weeks you don't notice any difference, the yogurt you are eating possibly does not contain enough acidophilus and bifidus bacteria. In that case, I suggest you try a probiotic supplement that contains these two types of bacteria. Many years ago, my wife had severe colic and digestive problems and a supplement containing acidophilus and bifidus had almost a miraculous effect on her digestive challenges.

The Hunza people eat yogurt regularly and so do most of the other cultures that have many centenarians including the Okinawa people, the Abkhazians, the Georgians and the Vilcabamba people from Ecuador. If most long lived cultures eat yogurt, why not copy them and live longer yourself. The yogurt you eat must contain the acidophilus and bifidus culture which have a dramatic effect on improving your stomach digestion.

Kefir and good bacteria for your stomach and to relieve stress

Kefir is a fermented milk product similar to yogurt, that originated in the Caucasus area of Russia where many of the people live to be a healthy and lively 100 years old. Kefir is made from kefir grains and fermented milk and has a more good bacteria than yogurt.

Dr Elie Metchnikoff, one of the first people to research kefir, was an immunologist who received the Nobel Prize in 1908 for discovering phagocytosis. He was amazed at the longevity of the people of Bulgaria and the Caucasus area of Russia where kefir was a staple food they consumed. Kefir contains good bacteria (probiotic), vitamin B12 and B1, vitamin K, calcium, magnesium, phosphorus and the amino acid trytophan which has a relaxing effect on the nervous system thus reducing stress. Regularly drinking kefir will result in relief of intestinal problems, remove flatulence, regulate bowel movements, assist in digestion of food, and generally improve health and longevity. I have recently discovered this astonishing food and I purchase kefir from my local health food store in the refrigerator at 4°C. I buy the Babushka brand and it costs $5.95 for 500 ml. You take about ¼ cup (62 g) per day which is a small investment in a longer, less stressful and disease-free life.

MORE ENZYMES=LONGER LIFE; LESS ENZYMES=DIE QUICKER

Dr Howell, in 1940, said that degenerative diseases such as arthritis were caused by a severe deficiency of enzymes. Raw foods contain many enzymes, however, cooking food above 48°C destroys all enzymes. If you eat mainly cooked foods you are using up your body's supply of enzymes. When the body gets to the point of enzyme deficiency, premature ageing begins and diseases such as arthritis occur. This was taken from an article from Roger French, the CEO of the Natural Health Society.

EATING ENZYME RICH FOODS	EATING COOKED FOOD
INCREASES YOUR LIFESPAN	DECREASES YOUR LIFESPAN

CHOOSE WISELY

Enzymes and your liver

How your liver works

Understanding the liver and how it works is very important for your future longevity and also to understand what foods can nourish and detox the liver when you have eaten the wrong types of food over a long period of time.

Your liver is designed to filter your blood from all the garbage such as bacteria, parasites and other harmful invaders. Do you filter the water in your swimming pool regularly? Of course you do, it is not wise to swim in dirty water full of garbage as you could pick up some dangerous diseases, right! You can easily change your swimming pool filter but you cannot change your liver when it gets full of rubbish. Lucky for you there are many enzymes that help your liver perform these life-saving functions. The amazing liver contains Kupffer cells which are have a special purpose to remove the garbage from your blood. Those of you who have major liver problems, I strongly recommend you read *The Liver Cleansing Diet* by Dr Sandra Cabot. She gives simple explanations and real cures.

A fatty liver

We love the tasty meats containing too much fat as well as other sources of fat. But we don't see the disaster taking place in our liver as a result of high fat consumption. It is wise to have a blood test at least twice a year to highlight the condition of your liver as well any other problems with your body. We are born with one body and we have the choice to take good care of it or to neglect and abuse it and suffer the consequences such as ill-health, disease, surgery to correct problems and a stay in hospital. Going to hospital could be your wakeup call from God. Either we choose to change our food habits or the universe will give us a jolt to shake our lives to improve our health.

A healthy liver and a longer life

We spend a lot of time trying to look after that super pump, our heart, and that is very important. We look at the mirror in the morning and try to improve our outward appearance to make us feel good and we need to do that. What about the hidden treasure inside our rib cage, the liver? It helps the heart by combining with bile to remove cholesterol. When we abuse our body by drinking too much alcohol, our liver is our only lifeline protecting our body from other damage. But the liver has its limits and cirrhosis of the liver can result from excess drinking of alcohol. Many years ago in one of my first jobs, a work colleague came to work with a yellow (or jaundiced) face and complexion indicating problems with his liver. This is a huge challenge to overcome. Whereas, a healthy liver means a longer and pain-free life.

Dandelion root and your liver

Recharge your liver by detoxing using dandelion tea. The Europeans and the Chinese have been using dandelion root tea for hundreds of years to heal the liver. We don't have a crystal ball to see what is inside our liver. Is it healthy and functioning well or is it getting overloaded with fats, pain killing tablets or chemicals hidden in the foods we eat? Common sense tells us that some regular maintenance on your liver by drinking some dandelion tea could be beneficial. Like many medicines, dandelion tea has a slightly bitter taste. Liver expert Dr Sandra Cabot discusses dandelion tea it in her book, *The Liver Cleansing Diet.* Herbalist Dorothy Hall recommends dandelion tea for obesity and liver problems and I strongly suggest you read her book, *The Natural Health Book.*

ACT   Action Creates Transformation

1. Eat more uncooked raw food such as fruit and vegetables as they contain essential enzymes. These enzymes in fruits and vegetables help save the body from making more of its

own digestive enzymes to assist in the digestion of food in the stomach. Professor Artturi Ilmari Virtanen, a Finnish biochemist and Nobel prize winner, showed that enzymes in uncooked food are released in the mouth when vegetables are chewed (refer to the excellent book *Raw Energy* by Leslie and Susannah Kenton).

2. Eat more yogurt especially those containing less sugar. Yogurt contains live bacteria like lactobacillus that add to the good bacteria in your stomach and help with digestion of food.

3. Drink more wheatgrass juice. A 30 ml shot of this enzyme rich juice is available from many juice bars, e.g. Boost Juice. This will improve your wellness level over a period of time and improve the enzyme level of your body. Remember, as we get older our enzyme levels start to drop. Most cultures that have great longevity, e.g. the Hunza people, eat enzyme rich food every day.

4. Regularly drink dandelion root tea to help cleanse your liver of toxins. This enables the liver to create more of the essential enzymes that the body needs to function at its optimum level.

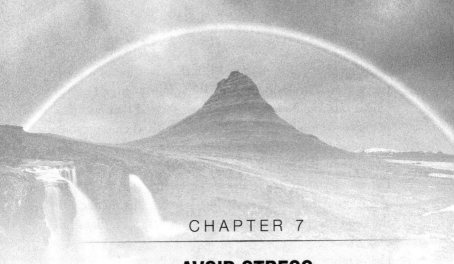

CHAPTER 7

AVOID STRESS

The more you focus on stressful things in your life, the more you attract more stressful events. As you change your thoughts to calming, peaceful and relaxing things in your life, the universe will send you more calming, peaceful and relaxing things.

Stress begins outside the body, it is an external invader that acts with stealth to slowly capture the nervous system and it feeds on your own anxiety to increase your blood pressure. Your sense of balance and how you perceive the world starts to change.

There is a common sense balance that should form your day, week and eventually your year. This includes time for love, time for work, time for family, time for eating healthy food, time for relaxing with family and friends, time for study to sharpen our brains, time for exercise, time for getting our finances together, time to laugh, time to look deeper into what God represents to us, time to reflect on our life and the lessons we need to learn and apply to our life, time to process stress in a different way, time to listen and learn, time to help others, time to look after ourselves, time to suffer so we can change ourselves, time to believe in a higher power that creates order in our world, time to believe in ourselves, time to lead and time to follow, time to study a garden and plant a seed and watch it grow and time to sleep and be rejuvenated.

Some questions to ask yourself about your life

How do you spend your time, are you focused too much on one area of your life and is this giving you stress? Are you focusing on the people you like or the people giving you trouble?

Could it be you are attracting more stress to you by your thoughts and actions?

Regarding your loving partner in life, do you focus on their good points or their bad points and why? Is it better to work on improving yourself first rather than your loving partner?

Why do you eat so much junk food, is it because the TV convinced you or was it your inner voice? Is the best time to start exercising now or after you have a heart attack?

Why are you running your life at 120 kilometres an hour and is it ruining other parts of your life? Do your emotions control you or do you control your emotions?

Sometimes the people around you are guiding you in the right direction but are you ready to listen? Are you spending enough time with your children? Are you spending enough time with your loving partner?

Instead of waiting for appreciation from other people, why not start to appreciate other people first? Do you give thanks to God for the things you have, rather than focus on what you have lost?

Types of stress

Sickness

Life-threatening sickness creates stress in your body and in your family. The emotions start to fire up. What will happen to me? Will I die? How will I work? How will I survive?

Sometimes, when we are faced with death or a loved one faces it, for the first time we start to look at what is really important in our life. A healthy body becomes very important. It is like an alarm bell is ringing inside of you. How did I get sick? It is not the time to blame other people for your sickness. You have control over the choices you make such as what you put in your mouth every day and the thoughts you dwell on, whether positive or negative. Is it your tasting tongue that controls you or your awareness of what are healthy foods that support your body and give you health?

Your wake up call to change your life can come in many forms such as cancer, heart problems, liver problems, gallstones, skin cancer, depression, kidney issues and many other challenges. Sickness means you need to change something about yourself. It is time to listen and be motivated to listen to the internal warning in the shape of sickness. Chances are somebody around you was prompting you to guide you in the right direction but you ignored those prompts.

Sickness leads to you thinking you are responsible in some way for this happening but you should look at this in a positive way which can lead to positive change. In contrast, a negative way of looking at is to ask, "Why me?" and beat yourself up about it which won't change anything.

Transformation begins when you make a decision to change your ways. The beautiful butterfly emerges with great struggle from its cocoon and it will never be the same again. As its wings dry, it takes a leap into a new world and soars into the air high above the flowers. This could be you soaring into a new world with a healthy body if you listen to the warnings your body is giving you. When you change, the world starts to change and you will see things around you that you never noticed before. This could be the beauty in your wife or the smile of a child and you will see more healthy people around you. The reason for this is that you have become a healthy person yourself.

You need to persist and to keep trying to make healthy choices. You might fail for one week and make too many bad choices but water, like persistence, wears away the rocky sea cliff and I believe you have what it takes to lift yourself up to a better way of life.

One advantage of suffering a life threatening illness and overcoming it is you will become much more compassionate to your family and friends and seeing your energy and zest for life they in turn will be inspired to change their lives. You have learnt a life lesson, that is, you are born with one body so take care of it and it will serve you well, but neglect your body and stress will follow you like a shadow. I hope the light is shining on you to eat healthy foods most of the time and your finely tuned instrument, your body, will be a dynamo of energy. Choose wisely what you put in your mouth.

Being overweight

Taking responsibility for your own actions is a starting point. Why am I doing this to myself? Cause and effect is a basic principle of life. It is my own hand that fed me the wrong type of food into my own mouth. Where did the term junk food come from? If you put junk into your body then you are slowly poisoning your own body. When you love your body you will take more care of your precious body. You love your wife or your husband, and you take care of her or him, right? Then, why are you not taking care of your God given body.

The answers to most mysteries lie within us. It could be we have low self-esteem or we are unhappy about some aspect of our life. It could be time to reflect on our life and start finding reasons why this happened.

When did this begin?

What triggered me to eat excessively? When did the habit of overeating start to get a hold on me?

Could the light bulb of a turning point in my life begin at this very moment?

We are digging deep for gold, not the type of gold that glitters but the nuggets of knowledge that will change your life. The present moment that you are reading this could be a decision time at the crossroads of your life. Keep going the way you are and it could be an early death, leaving your loved ones behind. Why not transform your life today and leave a legacy of a healthy body to inspire your wife or husband, your children and your close friends? There are millions of people who have defeated obesity around the world. Why not you? If other people can do it, you can too.

Life's battles are not always won by the strongest or the cleverest but instead it is the person who thinks they can change and applies persistence and determination and sets goals to climb their internal mountain. I believe in you and you can believe in yourself.

Financial stress

How do you handle money? Why do you have multiple credit cards? Do you plan your spending? Do credit cards help you to overspend leading to stress?

When we find ourselves in financial stress, chances are we would go to a financial expert. One of the first things they would ask us is to show them our budget. Well, do you have a budget?

There are two ways to handle your money:

1. Money comes in and money goes out. Where did the money go in the last year? This is the no plan approach leading to stress in the long term.
2. Written plan. This is the budget approach where money is allocated in advance each week for rent, food, electricity, fun etc. Planning your spending leads to peace of mind in the long term.

Which plan do you follow right now? Only you can change your life. Is it time to change your financial habits? Overusing credit cards and having no plan for spending, leads to stress while debit cards and a budget plan lead to peace of mind. Choose wisely for your future.

IF YOU FAIL TO PLAN, YOU PLAN TO FAIL

Author *Unknown*

Imagined stress

We give ourselves stress by imagining what might go wrong in our lives in the future. We are experts at worrying and stressing about what is going to go wrong in our lives. For example, we lose sleep thinking: How will I pay off my loans? What happens if I lose my job? What if my loved one dies? What happens if there is a recession? What happens if I can't pay the rent? What happens if I get sick and can't work?

I call this future gone wrong. The opposite of this is future gone right. Only you can control your own thoughts so please lead them in the right direction for your own peace of mind. One day as I left church, a priest said to me, "Inside of us we have two voices, the voice of the angel and the voice of the beast. Whichever you feed the most wins."

The past can be a source of stress if we are always thinking about events that happened in the past, for example, you had a car accident and you spent considerable time in hospital recovering from broken bones and the trauma of the accident which gave you much stress. You made a good recovery and it would be natural to talk about this event for a period of time after the accident. The time comes when you need to let go of this event so you can move forward in your life. An aeroplane travelling at 700 km an hour leaves turbulent air behind the plane and uses present time fuel to move the plane forward to its destination. We need to leave our problems behind us and live in the present moment so we can move forward in our life. We need to learn the lessons of the past and invest them in our future but leave the past behind.

The stress of fear

I have lived a long life and had many troubles, most of which never happened. – Mark Twain

Most of the things that we are afraid of never happen. Many years ago I was studying metallurgy and in my first year, my teacher asked me would a like to give a speech at the annual student speech night at the Institute of Metals. I said no as fear overtook me. I reasoned to myself that I had never spoken in public before and was worried about what the audience might say and I knew there were going to be many managers and CEOs present. A week later, an angel of courage must have landed on my shoulder and suggested I go for it so I approached my teacher and agreed to give the speech. On the appointed night, in addition to me, there were five other students giving speeches from other universities and TAFE colleges. I was quite nervous but I faced my fears and gave my speech. It wasn't the best speech of the night but the amazing thing that happened was many of the managers approached me and gave me encouragement to continue with my studies. In fact, this was a turning point in my life because, three years later, I found myself working in the same company, Hawker de Havilland, as one of the managers who had spoken to me that night.

Many times in your life, the fears that you have the courage to triumph over lead you to a better life. It is as if the universe sends you tests disguised as life lessons and if you can step out of your comfort zone and defeat those fears, you move forward to the next chapter of your life.

Stress at work

Do you love your job? When you love your job, you will experience less stress than if you hate your job. Even when you do love your work there may be times when you will have trouble meeting deadlines. You could experience personality clashes in dealing with some colleagues or most likely have too much work to do and not enough staff to handle the work load.

Ways in which to handle stress and to relieve stress

Talk to someone you trust

Talk to a friend or colleague or someone you trust about your particular situation and what you are struggling with. They need to be a good listener. A priest told me that when somebody has a major problem they need to unload the problem on somebody they can trust completely. Hopefully the person listening to the problem is not judgemental. Removing the problem off your chest has a way of removing tension from your body.

Physical activity

A good way to relieve stress is to regularly engage in physical activity such as working out at the gym, walking, yoga, Tai Chi, stretching to remove built up stress in neck and shoulders, playing sports, e.g. tennis, cycling, swimming, basketball etc. Experiment and find out what works for you.

Walking

Walking for 20 minutes three or four times a week is a great stress reliever. Simple walking helps the blood circulation, increases lung capacity and increases oxygen, giving a mood boost. Walking has a way of dissolving problems and while you are walking you often come up with solutions. The bigger the problem, potentially the further you could walk, within the physical limits of your body. When facing the biggest problems or the most stressful times in my life such as the loss of my father many years ago, I discovered walking helped me immensely to accept what had happened and deal with grief. Simple walking could be the prescription you need to change your life and reduce stress.

Breathing

Breathing is a natural part of life but how do you breathe? Most people breath with the top part of the chest. Diaphragm breathing means breathing from the bottom of the stomach and it relaxes the mind and the body. Many years ago when I was tutoring a high school student who was very nervous about her upcoming High School Certificate final exam, so I taught her the "Relaxing Breath", a breathing technique that involves breathing in to the count of 4, holding the breath to the count of 7 and breathing out to the count of 8. You breathe in through your nose using your diaphragm and breathe out through your nose. Do this for about 2 minutes. My student did pass her Higher School Certificate in second unit English and she thanked me for how relaxed she felt. You too can relax by using this technique when you are faced with stress at work or wherever else in life.

Yoga

The ancient practice of yoga, which combines stretching and toning exercises helps relieve the tensions that build up in our muscles when we experience stress. Professional athletes today, whether they play tennis, football, soccer or any other sport, practice stretching exercises before they compete in sporting events. Experience has proven that they suffer fewer injuries if they stretch and warm their muscles before playing sport. Yoga combines stretching and breathing exercises together that relax the mind, body and spirit. The Hunza people have been practicing yoga for many hundreds of years and considering their great longevity, we could learn a valuable life lesson from these peaceful and calm people.

Hatha yoga is one of the simplest types of yoga to begin your relaxation journey that could dramatically remove the tensions and stress from your life. Reading about this is a spark that helps you, I hope, to take action to transform your life. An investment of 15–20 minutes a day in yoga exercises will improve your blood circulation, relax your muscles, calm your nerves, increase your serenity and increase your energy and vitality. Breathing exercises are an important part of yoga and the ancient yogis call breath prana. This prana is a vital energy force that is built up in the body through correct breathing practice and it is literally a "life force" that can change your life. Yoga will improve your posture and as your posture improves your back pain will reduce and your neck, shoulder and scapula pain will start to disappear. Remember, yoga is not instant coffee, it takes time to get results. As you continue to practice yoga, slowly the stress will be eliminated from your body.

Tai Chi

Tai Chi is an ancient form of exercise that began in China. Today it is practiced by millions of people all over the world. Whether you are young or seventy years old, you will benefit from practicing Tai Chi, especially in reducing stress. For the last 15 years, I personally have practiced Tai Chi and these are the benefits I have experienced:

- Reduced stress
- Increased energy
- Peace of mind

- A focused mind
- Clear thinking
- Increased health
- Improved circulation
- Better sleep
- Healing hands (according to my wife).

The longer you practice Tai Chi, the greater the benefits especially increased energy, calm, peace of mind, better concentration and mental focus.

Have fun

How many times did you laugh today? The people who laugh the most are young children; they never seem to be depressed. I think we can all learn something about having fun from young children. A good hearty laugh reduces stress and the brain releases endorphins into the blood stream which give you that happy feeling. Endorphins are more powerful than morphine. That is why, some hospitals in Australia are inviting people like volunteers from the Starlight Children's Foundation to bring laughter and fun to the patients to help take their mind off their disease. We all need to bring out that "inner child" who is hiding inside of us. Think about children, all they want to do is have fun; they live in the PRESENT MOMENT, they don't think too much about the past and they don't worry about the future. They are mostly free of worry and anxiety. We all can learn a valuable life lesson from children.

How can you add fun and laughter into your life?

- Watch comedy movies such as Coneheads, or National Lampoons Christmas.
- Search for and spend time with people in your circle of friends who laugh a lot as they will automatically encourage you to laugh more. Remember, you slowly become like the people you hang around with.

- Visit a fun park like Lunar Park in Sydney and you are guaranteed to have a fun day.
- Find ways to make other people happy, give appreciation and encouragement to other people. What you do to other people comes back to you greatly multiplied; this is the Law of Compensation as described by Ralph Waldo Emerson, the great philosopher.
- Try fishing, where you can leisurely take in the rhythm of the waves and the smell of salt in your nostrils at the beach or the peaceful tranquillity of a river or lake. Enjoy it with some friends or take your loving partner with you. You will notice a lessening of the stress in your life.
- Go on a date with your partner to the cinema and treat yourselves with popcorn and a chocolate heart. This is fun and why not have a romantic dinner with your partner before the movie.
- Spend a weekend away with your loving partner close to the beach, there is no telling how much fun you might have.
- Laugh at yourself, don't take yourself too seriously. Many years ago I was teaching a group of high school students and I passed wind rather loudly. One of my students said, "I've never heard a teacher fart before!" Well, they laughed for what seems an eternity and I started to laugh myself. We tend to laugh at the expense of other people quite often, but the next time you make a mistake at work, instead of beating yourself up or running the tapes in your mind that evening, learn to laugh at your mistakes to ease the tension. Learn the lesson from the mistake, let go of it and look forward to a better day to come.
- Learn to dance with your partner, e.g. samba, Latin, hip hop etc. Get closer to your partner and start some slow dancing; add some fun and romance into your life.
- Enjoy a picnic lunch in the country with your partner. Inhale the fresh crisp country air, take along your favourite lunch, add some sparkle with a glass of wine, listen to some of your favourite songs and you are set for fun, laughs and romance.

Garry Gordon

Aromatherapy – Lavender oil

Discovery of aromatherapy

During the 1920s, a French chemist Rene-Maurice Gattefosse was working into the long hours of the night on a new perfume formula. He lost concentration while blending some essential oils and an explosion ripped through his laboratory and severely burned his arm. Seized with pain and stress, he looked around his laboratory and thrust his arm into the closest bowl of liquid. He felt immediate relief from the fires of pain and when he regained his senses he gazed in awe at the liquid that had saved his arm. It was lavender oil. The burn healed quickly with little pain and no scarring.

Rene devoted the rest of his life to the study of essential oils in healing. Aromatherapy is using essential oils derived from plants and herbs to heal the body by smelling the aromas.

Lavender oil to reduce stress

Lavender oil can be used to reduce stress by placing a couple of drops of lavender oil on your pillow case just before you go to sleep. Try it! In the workplace or at home add a few drops of lavender oil to some potpourri (dried flowers) in a small bowl and smell it often.

Headaches from stress can be relieved by applying one or two drops of lavender oil to your temples or the back of your neck. Remember, lavender oil is highly concentrated so you only need a few drops. Use a quality lavender oil for the best effect.

Peppermint tea

Peppermint is the main ingredient in most medications available from the chemist for flatulence and stomach disorders. Why not go directly to the source and buy some good quality peppermint tea bags. Boil some hot water, add one or two tea bags to your cup depending on the severity of your stomach pain, and pour the boiling water over it, and allow at least 3–4 minutes to let the peppermint infuse into the boiling water. My wife has been using this for many years and it most often gives a better result than over the counter medications. Many people experiencing stress feel pain in their stomach so, if that is your experience, try the healing effect of the amazing peppermint tea.

Chamomile tea

When stress stops you from sleeping well and you tend to "run the tapes in your head" of what happened at work try drinking chamomile tea. One hour before you go to sleep, put one or two teabags of chamomile tea in a cup of boiling water, let the infusion draw for at least 3–4 minutes and drink slowly. You will discover that you will have a better night sleep and feel rejuvenated in the morning.

Forgiveness

When stress is the result of someone harming you physically, emotionally or mentally, you have two choices: revenge which will take you down the dark side of the universe, or compassion which slowly leads to forgiveness that is the inner voice of the light within.

You cannot overcome the enemy until you have healed in yourself that which you find despicable in them – From an ancient Chinese text.

There are four kinds of forgiveness:

- The first is beginner's forgiveness for yourself. Many years ago I was in my third year of my Metallurgy Certificate and was preparing to sit for my final exam for that year. The teacher said to write down the day of the exam, the time and the place but foolishly I did not follow his instructions. I turned up the next Tuesday in my normal room at the usual time but nobody else was in the room. I started to panic a bit and went up one floor in the lift and then down one floor but I could not find my class. Unable to understand what was happening, in desperation, I walked rapidly to the main administration building to try and find the exam timetable. In my confused state of mind I could not find it and when a teacher came out of the staffroom, I asked him about my "metal forming" exam He disappeared into the staff room and five minutes later he with the news, "That exam was held yesterday". I was stressed out, wondering what will happen and after a restless night I made an appointment to see the principal the next day. I told him I had no excuse and I alone was responsible for turning up on the wrong day. He informed me that I would have to wait another year to do the exam again. The problem eventually turned into an opportunity because after talking to the principal I bought a diary and began to record important appointments in my diary. Strangely, after that I became very punctual and have not been late for a final exam since that fateful day. Also I forgave myself for the mistake and let go of it so I could move forward in my life.

- The second kind of forgiveness is beginner forgiveness for another person who has slightly wronged you in some way for example, the principal who told me I had to wait another year instead of allowing me to sit the exam again in the same year. I knew he was just following the rules of the TAFE college and that I was responsible for what had happened so there was no sense in blaming him for my mistake. Because of that, it was much easier to forgive the principal and turn it into a learning experience for me.

- The third type of forgiveness is advanced forgiveness for yourself when you break your own standards and values. Making mistakes and breaking our own rules is almost part of being human. When we break our own set of rules of what we value, we tend to feel shame and dwell on our own error of judgement. It is normal to feel some guilt and remorse for a period of time; however, we need to jump over our own self-imposed obstacle so we can move forward. We need to learn the life lesson and let go and release the event so we can move forward in our life.

- The fourth and most challenging type of forgiveness is advanced forgiveness for another person who has severely hurt us in some way which is something that happens to all of us at some point in our life. Deciding to take revenge or dwelling on the hurt for an extended period will lead to hate and travelling down the "dark side of the force". Jesus's prayer says, "Forgive us our trespasses (faults) as we forgive those that trespass (hurt) against us". Jesus's prayer did not say to make revenge against people who hurt us, that would mean perpetuating more evil but instead he says to forgive other people. to let go and release them from your mind and heart. Forgiving is all about removing the tapes in your mind and to stop replaying the events of hurt again and again like a movie in your conscience. It does not mean the other person did the right thing, but it helps *you* let go of the person and past event so that you will be the one with peace of mind. We all have a choice about what we focus on in our mind. When we focus on peace of mind then it is peace of mind that is growing in our mind and our world. On the other hand, if we focus on the hurts of the past then the universe tends to give us even more hurts to focus on. Choose wisely your focus because what you focus on the most will show up in your life, more and more. I hope you choose peace of mind.

Forgiveness is like sitting in your car and looking forward so you can see where you are headed. In contrast, when you spend too much time looking in your rear view mirror at what is behind you, it is like looking at past hurts most of the time and your life will not move forward while focusing on the past. The purpose of past events is to learn life lessons from them and invest what we have learned from those lessons in our future.

Many years ago, my wife and I attended a seminar about forgiveness. The leader of the seminar was Sister Margaret Scully, one of the wisest people I have ever met. She asked everybody to write down on a piece of paper the person and event from the past that has most hurt us. We then each ignited our piece of paper and put the burning papers into a large urn and watched as the smoke rose and our hurts slowly drifted away. Watching many people crying and cleansing themselves of past hurts, resulted in many people being healed on that amazing day.

Forgiveness technique

1. Write down on a piece of paper the person and event that has hurt you the most. Writing helps cleanse your heart and mind and removes it out of your system.
2. Burn the paper in the garden or anywhere safely. This symbolizes the letting go of the person and event. As the paper burns watch the smoke being released into the air. If you happen to cry at this time, your tears are like a safety valve that helps relieve the stress and tension that has built up inside you over this event.
3. Pray a silent prayer for that person, e.g. I now release that person and let them go and I wish them peace, love and harmony right now. Praying for them shows God and the universal laws that you have forgiven that person and are now moving forward in your life.

When you hold on to a person or event that has given you great trauma, you are continuing to give them power over you, They are not losing sleep over the event, you are. When you truly forgive them you become empowered to move forward in life. The stress of the past is finally released and you are filled with peace of mind.

If you want to live to be 100 years old, you need to remove as much stress from your life as you can, especially if the stress is created by you and your fears. Learn the lessons of wisdom from the Hunza people who walk at least ten kilometres a day to tend their orchards. Okay, you may not have an orchard to tend, but why not dare to change your life and reduce your stress levels by walking say one kilometre a day which could take 20 to 40 minutes. Your heart will pump more oxygenated blood around your body, your breathing will be deeper and your nervous system will slow down and you will feel an increase in energy, vitality and happiness. When you make this a habit it will work wonders in your life and the people around you will notice the difference. I have given you many techniques to reduce the stress in your life after much research on the subject.

You are the master of your destiny
now is the time to change your life and
have the courage to fire
up and get moving.

ACT Action Creates Transformation

1. Accept and recognize that you have stress in your life and have the courage to make a decision that it is YOU who needs to change something in your life, e.g. your attitude, your exercise discipline, your work/life balance, the type of food you eat, or your relationship with other people.

2. Attitude. If you spend most of your time complaining about the people you work with, your family, friends, what will happen is that the universe will give you more things to complain about. This is the "Law of Attraction". The opposite of complaining is gratitude and when you spend more time being thankful (counting your blessings), the universe will send you more things for which to be thankful. When you are ready to change your attitude to be more

thankful, the world around you will slowly change. The reason is because you have changed. Research says it can take about 21 days to change a habit. Each morning spend 5–10 minutes thinking of all the things for which you are thankful, e.g. your health, the food that you eat, your loving partner, your job, God for the gift of life, a roof over your head etc. Creating a gratitude journal is even more powerful as writing is a visual commitment to gratitude. Be daring and try it for three months and see how your life changes.

3. Work. If you love your job then you have discovered your purpose and you will have far less stress than if you hate your job. Stress at work can come from your work colleagues, the boss, customers, long hours, pressures of the job etc. If you have tried to change the people who you worked with and have been unsuccessful then you only have one choice left, that is to change your attitude and how you react to the people around you. This means practicing self-control through discipline of thoughts, words and actions. If you do not react to provocation, the other person will look for someone else to bother. Remember the law of "karma", that the people who make trouble for other people create much trouble in their own lives. The universe will always give like for like, so help other people and you will be helped, especially if you do not expect anything in return. Make trouble for other people and the universe will send you much more trouble in due time. Exercise more self-control, discipline can be learnt, and your peace of mind will help eliminate stress.

4. Exercise. When you have stress in your life, try walking for 20–30 minutes every day. The more stressful the situation the longer you can walk, but start slowly if you have not walked for a long period of time. The benefits are INCREASED ENERGY, less stress, deeper breathing meaning more oxygen in your blood and more vitality, releasing tension in the muscles and ligaments.

5. Yoga will increase the flexibility in your body and mind; you will become more serene, calm and balanced, and your spirit of peace, love and harmony will grow. Try hatha yoga or the "Five rites" by Peter Kelder. Who dares wins.
6. Practicing Tai Chi will result in much less stress, improved concentration, more energy, and a peaceful spirit.

I believe you can defeat stress.
*I would like to inspire and challenge you today to take **ACTION**.*

"Balance is the key to the universe."

Hugh Grech

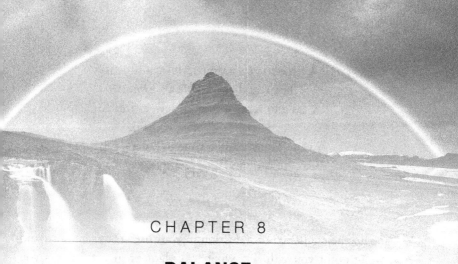

CHAPTER 8

BALANCE

What is balance?

The dictionary defines balance as a sense of proportion. The term 'common sense' means well balanced judgement. How many people do you know who have common sense? In life we meet many people who are intelligent, and as we grow older in years many of us develop more common sense. Experience teaches us and we develop common sense to overcome the problems we face in the struggles of life. Balance is what we seek when parts of our life become out of balance. For example, we may spend too much time and effort in the work part of our day.

> To everything there is a season, and a time
> to every purpose under the heaven
> A time to be born, and a time to die, a time to plant,
> and a time to pluck up that which is planted
> A time to kill, a time to heal, a time to
> break down, and a time to build up
> A time to weep, a time to laugh, a time to mourn, a time to dance
> A time to cast away stones, and a time to gather stones together,
> A time to embrace, and a time to refrain from embracing

> A time to get, a time to lose, a time to
> keep, and a time to cast away
> A time to rend, a time to sew, a time to
> keep silence, a time to speak
> A time to love, and a time to hate, a time
> of war, and a time of peace.

Ecclesiastes 3 from the Bible

Take up the challenge of reflection in your life. You were born and at some point you will die, what you plant or give to others you will eventually harvest, good things or bad things they will return to you from different people. There is a time to be sick, and a time to be healed, a time to be depressed and a time to build up your positive spirits again, a time to cry when overcome by stress, a time to laugh and be happy again, a time to mourn at the loss of a loved one, a time to dance and have romance. There is a time to remove certain material things not needed anymore, a time to gather more important things into your life, a time to hug people and a time to refrain from hugging, a time to receive, and a time to give, a time to keep the things that you love, and a time to get rid of the things that you hate, a time to divide, and a time to unite, **a time to keep silent and listen to the voice within**, and a time to speak and take action, a time to love, and a time to hate, a time for war and a time for peace.

A TIME TO FIND YOUR BALANCE.

How do you spend your day?

God gives us 24 hours to spend each day. How do we spend our day?

- Sleep –8 hours
- Work – 8 hours
- Eating meals, commuting to and from work, cleaning our bodies – 4 hours

- What do we have left? – 4 hours

Of this remaining 4 hours:

  o How much time do you spend listening and talking to your loving partner and your children?
  o How much time do you spend each day exercising your body, remember "use it or lose it"?
  o How much time do you spend thinking about other people's needs?
  o How much time do you spend exercising your mind by reading books that exercise your mind as part of life-long learning?
  o Laughing and having fun are an important part of a well-balanced life. What did you do to have fun today? The more time we spend making other people happy the happier we will be.
  o You are **mind, body and spirit,** are you investing equal amounts of time on each vitally important part of your vibrant life?

What part of your life do you get out of balance most often? Reflect on your present situation: are you spending too much time sleeping, working, cleaning your body, eating breakfast, commuting to work, or communicating with your family?

Most people might say they spend too much time at work, including checking work-based emails while at home. Are you experiencing stress because your life is out of balance? You created your day so why not take time to reflect on your day and start to make some changes to restore your balance. If you don't, you might be reflecting about this while recovering from a stress-related heart attack, nervous breakdown, cancer or other major illness in a hospital. If you want more peace of mind, plan today, say at 8 pm, what you are going to tomorrow, e.g. today is Monday at 8 pm so get your diary out and start planning what you are going to do on Tuesday in priority order. Remember, if you fail to plan you plan to fail.

List the five most important things you must do tomorrow, for example:

- 1. Eat a healthy vitamin charged breakfast to fire up your day.
- 2. 9 am – Meet with Catherine Ponder to work out the budget for the month.
- 3. 11 am – Speak to every member of the staff and say some encouraging things to them about their work and give them their schedule of daily activities.
- 4. 5pm –Ring your wife to tell her you are taking her on a romantic dinner date.
- 5. 8 pm – Plan your next day in advance.

The Law of Compensation – Essay by Ralph Waldo Emerson

"Polarity, or action and reaction, we meet in every part in nature, in **darkness** and **light**, **heat** and **cold**, in the **ebb** and **flow** of waters, in **male** and **female**, in the inspiration and expiration of **plant** and **animals**, in the systole and diastole of the heart, in the undulations of fluid and sound, in the centrifugal and centripetal gravity, in electricity, galvanism and chemical affinity. Superinduce magnetism at one end of a needle, the opposite magnetism takes place at the opposite end. If the **south attracts**, the **north repels**. To empty here, you must condense there. An inevitable dualism bisects nature, so that each is half, and suggests another thing to make it whole, as spirit, matter, **man, woman,** subjective, objective, in, out, upper, under, motion, rest, **yes, no.**"

When I first read this essay more thirty years ago something touched me like a bolt of lightning. The above passage is small extract of Emerson's essay. I dare you to find the full essay on the internet or borrow a book from the library about Emerson and read the complete essay (about 20 pages) and tell me what parts of this essay **touched your heart**. One year after you read the essay for the first time, read it again and I guarantee you will see different things in it that you did not see in the original reading.

Life is happiness and sadness, good times and bad times, love and hate, balance and out of balance, work and rest, peace and war, give and take, fear and courage, faith and doubt, going out and staying at home, and living and dying. There is a time to reflect and a **time to live in the present moment.**

The Wheel of Life

The wheel of life consists of

- Work
- Body –food and exercise
- Mental – exercising the mind (life-long learning)
- Spiritual – God and helping and contributing to the community
- Family and friends
- Sleep
- Fun and recreation
- Money and finances

How balanced is your wheel of life? When you have balance in your life, imagine turning a large wheel and your life will be mostly smooth. However, when one segment of the wheel extends beyond the outer circle then, as your wheel turns, you will hear clunk, clunk, clunk your life has become out of balance. When one element, such as work, takes up way too much time and energy and you experience stress and sickness then your family life will suffer and possibly you are not eating healthy foods so this can result in diseases in your body like cancer and heart attacks.

Reflect on your life right now. What parts of the wheel of life do you need to change? If you don't change then one day you might be reflecting on this in a hospital or in a coffin. I pray that you make wise decisions about things in the wheel of life that need changing for you and your family's future.

These are the parts of your life that might need changing, for example:

- WORK.   I have been spending 60 hrs a week at work and I feel tired, irritable and stressed out. When I get home I shout at my children and argue with my wife.
  I need to ....

- BODY.   I Eat mostly take away junk food that is mainly processed food. I rarely drink water and instead often drink soft drinks (acidic).
  I need to ....

  My main exercise is watching people on TV do exercises and thinking about walking in the evening after dinner but not actually doing it. I am overweight which eventually could lead to a heart attack.
  I need to ....

- SPIRITUAL.   I mainly think about myself and my wants and needs. My wife/ husband looks after the children. I go to the pub and discuss what is wrong with the world with my friends but don't take any action myself to improve the world and make it a better place to live. I think of God sometimes but only if I have a major disease or my wife or husband and children are very sick. I know I should help other people more and I gossip too much and should appreciate other people more instead of criticizing them behind their back. When I die, what would God say about how I lived my life?
  I need to ....

- MENTAL. I exercise my mind by watching TV and reading newspapers and gossip magazines. I have some friends who improve their minds by doing courses at TAFE, university and online study. They are always reading books to improve themselves.
I need to ....

- FAMILY AND FRIENDS. I spend so much time at work I don't have much time for my family and friends. Maybe I should chill out and take my wife/ husband and family to the cinema and accept more invitations to party with my friends.
I need to ....

- SLEEP. I love to stay up late and watch my favourite sports show and also watch movies until late. Usually, I get about 5 hours sleep each night and I can't concentrate at work the next day. I make silly mistakes at work and have no energy. Most of my friends get about 8 hours sleep each night and are happy and content in their jobs.
I need to ....

- FUN AND RECREATION. I am so tired from work and lack of sleep that on my days off I spend most of the time sleeping and watching TV. Most of my friends have a drive in the country on the weekends and attend parties and go out on dates with their wife/ husband.
I need to ....

- MONEY AND FINANCES. When I go shopping I love to use one of my four credit cards and I don't seem to be able to pay off my credit card within 30 days of receiving my statement. I currently owe $4,000 on my credit cards and the balance I owe seems to grow every month. My friend Warren says, why not start a written budget like small business people do when they operate their business. Warren only has debit cards and he has a written budget for the last 10 years; he always seems to be calm and relaxed when it comes to finances.

I need to ....

The wheel of life has 8 parts – Reflect on each part

Reflect on each part of your life and rate yourself as to how happy and satisfied you are with each area of your life from 1 to 10.

For example:

- WORK 5/10 Comment ....I spend way too much time at work and I don't love my job and find it to be a hard grinding job.
- BODY 3/10 Comment ....I am overweight because I eat too much junk food and I rarely exercise and have low self-esteem.
- MENTAL 4/10 Comment.............I spend little time improving myself and I know I need to change.
- SPIRITUAL 2/10 Comment .... Mostly, I only think about myself. My wife/ husband goes to church and spends a lot of time helping the local community and is always so happy. Perhaps it is me who needs to change.
- FAMILY AND FRIENDS 6/10 Comment..........I spend a lot of time with my friends drinking beer in the pub. It is time to spend more quality time with my wife/ husband and family so I need to get my priorities and values in the right order.
- SLEEP 7/10 Comment ....Through the week I get about 5 hours sleep each night but on the weekend I make up for this with extra sleep. It is time to turn off the TV at 10 pm and be committed to a good night sleep, so when I wake up at 6 am in the morning I know that I have slept 8

hours and will feel focused, alert and energetic and ready to enjoy my working day.
- FUN AND RECREATION 5/10 Comment ……… Working way too many hours at work has resulted in a lack of fun and excitement in my life. My wife/ husband is right and it is time to reduce my working hours and increase the fun, excitement and romance in our lives.
- MONEY AND FINANCE 3/10 Comment ……….It is time to follow the wise advice of my friend Warren and slowly over time pay off all of our credit cards. I need to draw up a plan of action in the form or a written budget so eventually we can cut up our credit cards and only have debit cards so that we will live within our weekly budget.

We need to monitor the wheel of life once a month, for example, let us do it on the first day of the month.

___/___/_____ (*record the date*)

- WORK 5/10
  I need to change…………………………………………………

- BODY 3/10
  I need to change…………………………………………………

- MENTAL 4/10
  I need to change…………………………………………………

- SPIRITUAL 2/10
  I need to change…………………………………………………

- FAMILY AND FRIENDS 5/1
  I need to change…………………………………………………

- SLEEP 7/10
  I need to change…………………………………………………

- FUN AND RECREATION 5/10
  I need to change...

- MONEY AND FINANCES 3/10
  I need to change...

A review of the wheel of life needs to be completed 12 times a year. This is part of life-long learning. When you demonstrate a big improvement in one part of the wheel of life, e.g. you improve BODY from 3/10 to 7/10, why not reward yourself for this achievement by taking your partner out to the cinema and a romantic dinner. If you fail to reward yourself, who will reward you? By rewarding yourself, your subconscious will pick up the connection and help you to improve other parts of the wheel of life.

Your doctor monitors your blood pressure and hopefully you have a blood test every six months or so to discover if you have any diseases in your body. Why not take time to monitor important parts of the wheel of life so you can help prevent stress, heart attacks and other major stress related-diseases growing in your body. The more balanced your life, the longer you will live and you will be reducing the chances of being put in a nursing home when you are in your late sixties or seventies. If you want to be more energetic, loving, calm, stress free, vibrant and romantic, reflect on getting your wheel of life in balance. You are master of your destiny by how you live your life every day, apply the wisdom of the wheel of life so you discover peace, love and harmony in your life every day.

Examine your wheel of life and address any imbalances

Often in life we can be very quick to look at the weaknesses in other people but are very slow to take action to try to improve our own weaknesses. Let us right now examine our own wheel of life and take responsibility for our weakness.

When you have completed your own wheel of life, take a look at the area that is the weakest.

For example, a Body Score of 3/10 might be your weakest area.

Steps for changing yourself to increase your Body Score.

1. Accept you need to exercise more

    Create a plan for exercising. Buy a large planning type calendar with plenty of space for the individual days of the month. Place it in a prominent place in your house/unit, e.g. on the fridge door or kitchen wall. Make space in your week for exercising

    e.g. Walking:

    > Monday 7 pm to 7.30 pm, Tuesday 7 pm to 7.30 pm, Wednesday 7 pm to 7.30 pm

    e.g. Yoga/Tai Chi/lifting dumbbells.

    > Choose one of these activities and take dynamic action by DOING IT!

    > Monday 7.30 pm to 8 pm, Tuesday 7.30 pm to 8 pm, Wednesday 7.30 to 8 pm

2. Monitor (keep score) – place a large tick or write the word VICTORY on your calendar plan when you successfully complete each exercise session.
3. Reward yourself – at the end of each week when you are successful with your weekly exercise plan, purchase something that gives you pleasure, e.g. clothes, a DVD, a ticket to the cinema or take your partner out on a romantic date.

4. Be committed to your plan – they say it takes about 28 days to change a habit. Be master of yourself by being motivated to change your wheel of life, for example, in the area of exercise. I believe you can do it, have faith in yourself and never give up on yourself.

In most cultures with greater longevity, the people are balanced

Most people from cultures with greater longevity are masters of their habits and have faith in themselves. These characteristics are reflected in the Hunza people of northern Pakistan, the Okinawa people of Japan, the Vilcabamba people of South America, the Abkhazians of Russia and the Ikarian people of Greece, all of which have many of their people living to be 100 years old. These people are balanced with very few signs of excesses in any areas of their life.

These cultures do not overeat and have very few overweight people compared to the rest of the world. They all walk long distances every day and have no cars, trains or buses. That is why they are physically strong with few signs of heart disease and other major diseases. They are emotionally balanced with close family ties. They exercise their bodies every day and go to bed early and get up early. They relax practicing yoga and spend as much time with their family as they can.

What about your life, how much time do you spend exercising? How much time do you spend with your family? Can you see the lessons we need to learn from these people and practice them in your own life?

These people love what they do for work in their country and work is fun for these cultures. They never retire they are life-long learners! In the rest of the world, statistics show that in the first two years of retirement many people die because possibly they start watching too much TV and they don't exercise enough. Their life-long habits of eating too much junk food and too much acid forming meat catch up with them and they suffer joint problems (too much acid forming meat) and other diseases linked to their bad food habits. It is not easy to look at ourselves in the mirror and let go of our pride and realise that the food we put in our mouth every day is shaping our lives for abundant health or disease, depending upon what we eat every day.

The people of these cultures with greater longevity are generally easy going, happy people, loving, friendly, intelligent and energetic, possibly because the natural unprocessed foods they eat act like a super fuel that balances every part of their life. Imagine if you and your children could learn and practice these habits to change your life from disease-prone to disease-free. What an exciting, happy, energetic life you would have!

For some reason, people of these cultures don't seem to have as many vices as the western cultures, with no drug addicts, very little crime, and very few overweight people. They do drink their own home made wines but do so in a moderate balanced way. They eat very little meat and exhibit very little disease. They have strong family values so there is very little crime. It looks like their sense of moderation or balance leads these people to a greater wisdom to look after their body, mind and spirit and take great care of their family.

When people find peace, love and balance inside themselves, then they will discover peace, love and balance in the world on the outside. May God help you discover a balanced life inside you and in your world.

ACT   Action Creates Transformation

1. Today, start creating your wheel of life.
2. Take ACTION and have the courage to look at your weaknesses in you wheel of life.
3. Make a plan to improve your greatest weakness. Remember, it is only **you** who can change your life but ask your partner

to help you and to motivate you. ACT on your plan and other people will notice the changes in you.

4. You also have strengths in your wheel of life. It is time to recognize and appreciate your own strengths and slowly you will also appreciate the strengths of your loving partner, your family, your friends and your colleagues at work. Appreciation of other people changes their lives and they in turn will start to appreciate their own family and friends. Gratitude for other people can change the world one person at a time and create more balance.

5. Spend more time in restful sleeping and less time late at night watching TV or surfing the internet.

6. Enjoy more quality time bonding with your family and less time doing overtime at work.

7. Observe your children and their sense of fun and how they laugh. Create more ways to find laughter and fun in your life.

8. Balance is about moderation in all things and focusing on the long-term important values and beliefs in your life.

There are three things that last forever,
faith
hope
and
love.
The greatest of these is love.

The family is created in love.

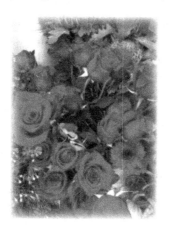

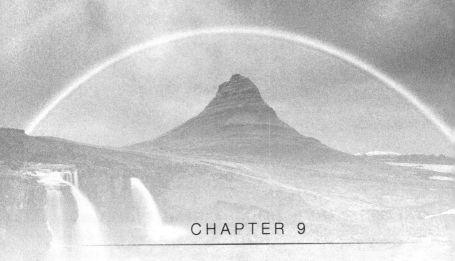

CHAPTER 9

FAMILY AND COMMUNITY

Most of us have been fortunate in having a mother and father who loved us and guided us, especially in our younger growing years. But not everyone has come from a happy family background and some people have had a very difficult and sad family life. If that is your experience, don't let your past sad experiences continue to affect your present life now. The past is done, let it go. You create your life today one thought at a time, one emotion at a time, one spoken word at a time and one action at a time. If you need help to leave the past behind, then ask for it. It is okay to ask for help, for example, from your GP or an qualified counsellor. Seek out the help you need to be free of past experiences that are stopping you from moving forward.

Let us focus on building a happy family, today, in the present moment. You are not perfect and your family is not perfect so how about you make a plan to build a happier, more fun-filled life and become a giver in your relationship with your family. All families have challenges, difficulties and stresses at different stages of life. If life was all roses, we would not have balance. When we overcome our challenges and stresses, we can appreciate the good times more and also be empathetic to understand the challenges other people face in their lives. Then, when other people come to us with their challenges, we will listen more intently to what they are saying, as we too have faced our own difficulties,

Cultures around the world that have many 100 year old citizens have strong family values such as

- Unconditional love
- Respect
- Trust
- Communication
- Always help each other (unselfish).

Relationships and family

Two individuals fall in love with each other and after a courting period and much romance, they marry each other. They become a family and their love is spiritual, mental, emotional and physical. Eventually, the first child is born and this builds another dimension to the relationship.

Forming a loving healthy relationship requires give and take, tolerance, persistence, a listening ear, and patience and understanding through the challenges that happen as the relationship grows and matures.

Sharing values (priorities) or beliefs about

- Love
- Spirituality
- Respect
- Honesty
- Trust
- Integrity
- Commitment

Actions and Activities

These values will lead to actions and activities such:

- Sharing loving moments with each other
- Saying "I love you" to each other every day
- Talking (communicating) with each other every day
- Listening to each other with focus on the other person
- Romancing each other, e.g. flowers, date nights, small gifts to each other and loving embraces
- Touching each other
- Holding hands
- Appreciating each other more rather than complaining about each other
- Sharing the work load at home as well as looking after the children
- Exercising with each other
- Openly communicating about money and setting budgets, e.g. 80% of couples divorce over money issues so this is important
- Accepting the strengths and weaknesses of each other
- Dwelling more on your partner's good points and less on their faults because we are all human, therefore, husband and wife will both have their faults
- Being committed to a life-long relationship and to forgiving each other when arguments develop
- Saying "Sorry". Sorry is a one of the hardest words to say but it leads to kissing and hugging to restore the relationship.

The four "diamonds" of a healthy marriage relationship

1. *Love*

   A healthy plant needs sunshine, water, and contact with fertile soil. A healthy marriage needs kind words spoken to each other every day, e.g. "I love you". We need to flow into the present moment and let go of the past and plan for the future, committed to each other through the good times and the bad. We need to romance each other, touch each other, hug each other and be spontaneous with each other.

We need to forgive each other when we upset each other and let go of that and be in the present moment again. Many of the problems in a relationship stem from dwelling on upsets that occurred in the past and worrying about what might happen in the future, e.g. loss of job and being unable to pay the mortgage or other "imagined" fears. We need to live in the present moment like a young child who is not concerned with the past or what might happen in the future, except at Christmas. A child lives in the present moment and we can learn a valuable lesson from a young child, as they laugh a lot and just want to have fun and be loved.

Love is patient, love is kind, love is respectful, love is accepting the other person just the way they are today. There are three things that last forever, faith, hope and love, but the greatest of them all is **love** (adapted from 1 Corinthians 13 from the Bible).

2. *Respect*

Speak about and appreciate the good points of your marriage partner and spend less time complaining about your partner. Get to know and understand the values and the family life that they experienced as they were growing up and realize that their experience will not be identical to your own.

Consider and respect your partner's ideas, feelings and personality (read *Personality Plus* by Florence Littauer to help you understand yourself, your partner and the people around you). Respect their opinion even when you don't agree with them.

Accept your marriage partner just the way they are.

3. *Trust*

Be a trustworthy person and keep your promises, those little promises as well as the big ones. Follow the rules of marriage.

Be open and honest when communicating with each other in private, but clearly understand what needs to be kept between the two of you and what can be shared with others.

Be the first to say sorry to diffuse a disagreement and get back to trusting each other. When trust is temporarily lost or either side, it can take work to bridge the gap so do not delay in rebuilding bridges.

4. *Communication*

Take time to talk to each other every day. When life is busy, stressful or difficult, it is even more important to take time to connect and communicate openly with other. Make allowance and listen more when your partner is sick or suffering in some way.

Spend time looking for the strengths in your partner rather than focusing too much on their weaknesses. Regularly, tell them what you appreciate about them.

Have fun with each other and have regular romantic dates with each other.

Conflict resolving skills

In every relationship, conflict is inevitable so developing your conflict resolution skills is essential for a healthy ongoing relationship. Don't let conflict go unresolved or it will build up and create a bigger problem and bring disharmony to your relationship and family.

- Define the problem clearly
- Both need to agree what the problem is
- Brainstorm together all possible solutions
- Say what changes each of you will personally make to arrive at a solution
- Summarise the solutions and act on the ones you both agree on

POEM

A good marriage must be created
In the art of marriage the little things, are the big things
It is never being too old to hold hands
It is remembering to say, "I LOVE YOU", at least once per day,
It is never going to sleep angry,
It is having a mutual sense of values and common objectives,
It is standing together, facing the world,
It is forming a circle of love that gathers in the whole family.

Author *Unknown*

Community

What is a community and what are the benefits?

A community is a group of people with a common interest. For example, if you love fishing then why not join a fishing club. The benefits are that you will mix with people who have a great knowledge about how and where to catch fish. You will extend your circle of friends and each new person you meet, besides your common interest in fishing, will polish a part of your character that you didn't know you had. Inevitably, they will tell you stories about their life struggles as well as their struggles to catch fish. Meeting new people is getting out of your comfort zone and learning more about other people's experiences in life. When I started volunteering, I joined a community of volunteers and I learnt so many things about the struggles other people face and the people God sends to improve the situation for them.

When you join a community you will meet people from other cultures who will tell you about their families and communities in their countries. For example, some may have lived in mountain villages and tell you stories about life surviving in remote areas with no supermarkets where they grow their own food and survive by helping each other, not competing with each other. Yes there are many lessons to learn when we communicate with people from other cultures and you will learn there are many ways to grow and cook food that are different from your ways.

We are blessed in Australia to have many different cultures from all over the world. The Italians taught us how to cook the best pizzas, to enjoy the pleasures of gelato ice cream and about the importance of hard work and having a close family. Vietnamese immigrants introduced us to their noodle dishes and their unique style of cooking as well as highlighting the importance of family and education. The Greeks taught us about Greek salad and Greek yogurt that help us live a longer life and about having strong family values. Japanese immigrants taught as how to eat sushi and seaweed that gives us a longer life and helped us to learn to respect each other and not to talk so much but to listen more. Immigrants from the Philippines taught us how to smile and love music, singing and the importance of family.

There are many other cultures I have not mentioned, but the point is we either learn from other cultures their "lessons of life" or complain about the minority that spoil it. True wisdom is about learning from others. As the parable in the Bible says, I complained about the splinter in the other person's eye but failed to see the log in my own eye.

You become more broad minded when you mix with other cultures and accept them the way they are. Remember, other people have families just like you and there is only a small minority with extreme views. Open your mind and your heart to people from different countries and cultures. Remember, there are seven beautiful colours in a rainbow so let us see the rainbows in the people of other countries and cultures. It is better to light a candle and bring light that can eventually create a rainbow rather than dwell in the darkness of what is wrong with the other person.

Common interests form communities and some of our outstanding business leaders started out in communities. For example, Dick Smith early in his life was a boy scout and more recently has helped The Smith Family by making substantial donations to this wonderful organization that has changed many lives through the work they do to help families in need.

Community connections of cultures known for their longevity

The Hunza people of northern Pakistan have strong family ties and they extend the family into the local community. They share the only real resources they have, that is the food they grow and helping other people tend their orchards through their shared skills, especially when other families lose loved ones in their families.

The Okinawa people from Japan have strong social networks even when they are 80–90 years old. In the amazing book, *The Okinawa Program*, the authors Bradley J. Willcox MD, D. Craig Willcox PhD and Makoto Suzuki MD talk about the friends and networks, and interests and passions that help us reach a healthy old age. If you don't have these ingredients in your life at this time, first take comfort in the fact that you are not alone – the Mayo Clinic tells us that nearly half of all Americans report that they don't have enough close relationships.

Church community

A church is where we go to love and worship God and to meet other spiritual people and share with them our experiences. There are no perfect people at church only God is perfect. We are all mind, body and spirit and as we grow in years we start to realize that life is also about helping other people. The more we help other people, it is as if the spirit of God grows within us and we become happier people.

We slowly become like the people we associate with and as we spend more time with spiritual people we tend to become more spiritual. Whereas, if we spend time with criminals we slowly take on the characteristics of criminals. We become magnetized by the people we spend the most time with. As the old saying goes "birds of a feather flock together".

Volunteering community

Last year, I spent about six months volunteering as a support worker with Share Care, a not-for-profit organization that looks after disabled children. Many of these children have challenging behaviours that they were born with. I met some outstanding volunteers and also the Share Care employees who showed so much, love, encouragement, patience, and kindness to these disabled children and helped them to have fun. I sensed that many of these children were brilliant in some ways but could not quite communicate this to the outside world. This was a very rewarding experience for me to try to understand how this group of people live with their own challenges.

It gives you a different perspective when we have a few minor challenges in our world. In trying to understand other people, we get to understand ourselves more and become more broad minded and, most importantly, more accepting of other people just the way they are.

How to find the right volunteer community for you

Choose a community that is close to your heart. For example, if you have lost a loved one through cancer, stroke, heart attack etc., why not join a support group connected to one of those diseases and give some of your time to support the friends and families so that you can share your experiences and the coping methods you used to get through those challenging times. Helping other people overcome their challenges is also a way for you to process and slowly let go of some of the anguish and difficulties you had when dealing with the sufferings of a loved one close to you.

Helping other people by volunteering your time and effort has a way of affecting your future. Remember, what goes around comes around. The world is like a mirror and when you give of your time, talent or treasure, it will come back in some other ways, especially if you give with no intention of receiving something back. The universe can tell the intention of the giver.

There are many charitable organizations such as Catholic Mission, House With No Steps, Kids with Cancer Foundation, Vision Australia, and Meals on Wheels, where you can donate your time, treasure or talent so that you can make a difference in the world. Remember, you have been supported by your family, friends and others at different times in your life and it is important not to forget these people as well. It is good to extend this to supporting and helping other communities. You have a certain measure of success in your life, so could this be the time to give back to the community that you live in so that others may experience your generosity?

Volunteering is also a way for younger and older members of the working community to learn new skills that can be utilized in your job or a future job. We live in changing times, whether you are a farmer, labourer, a factory worker, a business owner, a teacher, a web designer or you work in customer service. By donating some of your time to a volunteer organization, you can learn new computer skills, customer service techniques, telemarketing skills on the telephone, accounting skills, Information Technology and many other skills. You could also gain some real life experience on the job in a new area you want to work in, which you can add to your resume or CV. Recruiters can be attracted to job seekers who show some character by volunteering their time to make a difference in their community and at the same time gain experience in a skill the company is looking for.

It is when you step out of your "comfort zone" that the real learning takes place and you can also make a real difference in the world and the world of others who need your help desperately.

Art community

If you are a creative person who loves painting, drawing, photography, creating jewellery, writing poetry or any other artistic interest, how about joining a group of people with similar interests? Joining a community that reflects your interests will inspire you to develop your gift more so that you get inspired by people in the group and you in turn you will inspire others. Who dares wins. It is time to get out of your cave and explore and develop relationships with other people of similar interests.

Fitness community

Regular exercise is one of the secrets of long-lived and disease-free people groups. When are you going to begin a regular exercise program, while you are alive or will you wait too long?

Join a gym and let other people motivate you in your journey to a more vibrant and energetic lifestyle. It is time to transform your life from a couch potato watching too much TV and start to lose weight, increase your self-esteem and become a ball of dynamic energy.

Join a yoga class and learn about diaphragm breathing to get more energy into your body and to make your body more flexible. Yoga is an approach to exercise that is the opposite of the Western world approach to exercise. Yoga postures relax and stretch the body, releasing stress from within and strengthening the internal organs. My good friend Bruce Richards told me that if you practice yoga for at least three months, you will notice a big difference in your body and your energy levels. Remember, with any new exercise program start slowly as the body takes time to adjust to the different postures. Yoga will ensure that your heart will be pumping more efficiently with less stress and your bloodstream will carry more oxygen and give you more energy. Gradually, your back will become more flexible and your whole body will enjoy more flexibility. You will also reduce the chances of aching joints as long as you eat more alkaline forming foods, e.g. fruits and vegetables and less acidic forming food, e.g. meat. You need to help your body with discipline as well. The uric acid crystals that form in your joints and give you pain come from an excess of acidic forming foods eaten over a long period of time. Fruit and vegetables don't contain uric acid. Discipline of mind, body and spirit will help you live a longer life.

> To understand others is to have knowledge
> To understand oneself is to be enlightened
> To conquer others requires strength
> To conquer oneself is even harder

Lao Tze

Join a Tai Chi class as Tai Chi is one of the most gentle forms of exercise but when practiced for at least three months, it will sharpen your concentration, improve your memory, increase flexibility, reduce stress levels, create a calm and serene spirit in you and most importantly increase your positive energy levels. I have been practicing Tai Chi for at least 10 years and I know from experience it will change your life and you will become a more dynamic person with reduced stress levels as you become more serene and calm in your spirit. Change begins in your life when you change!

Garden community

When you plant a seed in the soil you nourish it with water and fertiliser and the sun provides the heat and energy to help germinate the seed, until after many days a plant slowly emerges from the soil. You can create a beautiful flower like a rose or perhaps grow a fruit tree in your backyard for a future harvest of oranges, apples, avocados, mandarins or any other of your favourite fruits.

You can cultivate a garden in your backyard or if you live in a unit why not grow flowers or vegetables in a garden pot. You can harvest organic food for your breakfast, lunch or dinner as long as you don't use poisonous sprays on your lovely vegetables and fruit.

Gardening is a great hobby and you can join a group of people with similar interests. For example, a friend of mine is a member of an Orchid Society. Or perhaps you could join a bonsai society to learn the Japanese secrets of cultivating these amazing miniature trees.

The Hunza people from northern Pakistan, the Okinawa people from Japan, and the Vilcabamba people from South America are all known for their longevity and they all grow their own food with no poisonous chemicals. Their supermarket is their own garden and they dry some of their food for use during winter. All of these cultures have no refrigerators or freezers but instead eat fresh produce out of their own orchards and gardens.

Gardening gives you creativity, exercise, peace of mind, calmness and helps reduce stress. When are you going to start your own garden and also join a garden community to help ignite your passion for the beauty of gardening?

Who dares wins. You win happiness, joy and abundant health!

ACT   Action Creates Transformation

1. Spend more time talking and having fun with your family and children. This last week how much time every day did you spend with your family and children?
2. Each day say I LOVE YOU to your loving partner and children at least twice every day.
3. Spend time today loving yourself by taking care of your mind, body and spirit. What did you do today to take care of yourself?
4. Did you join a community that has similar interests to you, e.g. gym, yoga, religious, garden, art, volunteer, cooking, fishing or public speaking (e.g. Toastmasters International)?
5. When you change, the world changes. Are you ready to change?

*Who created the universe with galaxies,
stars and planets ...?*

*Two people looked out of the same
window, one looks at the stars
the other looks at the mud.*

What do you see?

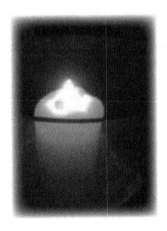

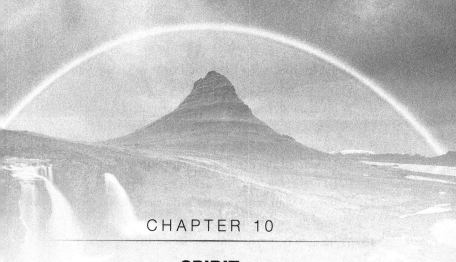

CHAPTER 10

SPIRIT

We all have different beliefs and different ideas about God and about spiritual things. For some, including many of those who have lived long lives, the spiritual element of their lives is extremely important, whereas, for others it is not something to which they devote much time or thought.

In this book, we have looked at many facets of life that affect how long we live, from looking after our physical bodies—what we eat and drink, and movement and exercise—to our attitude and mental health and also our social wellbeing in the context of family and community. The spiritual element is another facet of our lives that can have a significant effect on our longevity.

So, whether you believe in God or not, or whatever your religious beliefs are, please take time to seriously consider and answer these questions.

1. Who are you?
2. Where did you come from before you were born?
3. Who designed your mind, body and spirit?

4. What lessons of life have you learnt so far on planet earth?

5. Who created the universe?

6. Who created the stars?

7. Where do you go when the physical body dies?

8. Who created the first molecule of water?

9. Who started the earth spinning on its axis?

10. Why is there so much order in the universe?

11. What are your human gifts and where do they come from?

12. Where do positive emotions come from?

13. Where do negative emotions come from?

14. What are miracles and where do they come from?

15. Who was the first human being and who gave birth to that person?

16. Why is there a rainbow?

17. Who created colours? Why are there different colours?

18. Who made the first plant seed and where did it come from?

19. Where did the elements on the periodic table, e.g. oxygen, potassium, iron, come from?

20. How does a seed know when to germinate?

21. How does a deciduous tree know it is autumn and to start dropping its leaves?

22. Who created the oceans?

23. Who put the fishes in the first sea?

24. Where does love come from?

25. Who created the first fruit?

26. Who created the first vegetable?

27. Who created light?

28. Where does creativity come from?

29. Why do we age?

30. Where do inventions come from?

31. Where do the human gifts come from, e.g. painting, poetry, writing, playing a musical instrument and the gift of healing?

32. Who designed the human organs in the first human and who put blood in their body?

33. Who designed a cloud?
34. Where did Ralph Waldo Emerson's wisdom come from?
35. Who designed the five senses, i.e. sight, hearing, touch, taste and smell?
36. Where does truth come from?
37. Who designed the human heart?
38. Where does intuition come from?
39. What is light and who created the first light?
40. What is temptation and where does it come from?
41. Who created the first language and who taught the people to speak that language?
42. Where did gravity come from?
43. Where does wisdom come from?
44. Who created the first musical instrument and who taught that person to make it?
45. Why are there only seven colours in a rainbow and why can you not find the end of the rainbow?
46. How does a seed under the soil know to grow up and not down or sideways?
47. Why is there silence in space?
48. Who created the vacuum in space?
49. When you die where does your human spirit go?
50. Who created love?

In the journey of life of how to live to be 100 years old, we are all moving slowly to the light to be closer to God or we are moving closer to the darkness and the abyss. We are not perfect but the actions we take every day will determine our future.

The food we eat, the thoughts we cultivate, the exercises we practice, our life-long learning strategies, our methods in dealing with stress and our daily disciplines and habits are creating our future. I believe you can make the changes in your life to make a healthy, energetic and exciting life for you and your family.

ACT   Action Creates Transformation

1. Please complete the 50 questions and reflect on God and the meaning of life.
2. Are you moving close to the light of God or moving closer to the darkness?

FINAL WORDS

The writing of this book was completed on Valentine's Day, 14th of February, 2016 and I dedicate this book to my wife for her patience, endurance, faith and love.

In the journey of life, we all have our struggles and eventually the rain stops and a beautiful rainbow emerges like a caterpillar transforming into a butterfly.

I hope in your struggles in health I have opened your heart and mind to be touched by some of my research into the mysteries of how some cultures like the Hunza people from northern Pakistan, the Okinawa people from Japan, the Vilcabamba people from South America, the Ikaria people from Greece and the Georgian people from southern Russia manage to have so many people in their cultures that have solved the mystery of how to live to be 100 years old.

I thank you God for inspiring me in this seven year adventure to inspire other people to live a longer, happier, energetic and disease-free life.

I sincerely hope you live to be 100 years old and fill your heart with peace, love and harmony.

ACT   Action Creates Transformation

1. Study carefully all of your answers to the 10 chapters and try to take actions every day that will lead you to a long, healthy, happy, vibrant and inspired life.

*The end is the beginning of
a new life for you.*

*We hope you live to be 100 years
old and fill your heart with
peace, love and harmony.*

Take some time to read through the quotes and statements below and listen to the whispers from God to remind you of what we have talked about in this book. Now you have the knowledge, it is time for you to take action. You are the only person who can make the changes needed to inspire you to live to be 100 years old.

CHAPTER 1 – ACID /ALKALINE FOODS

The doctor of the future will combine traditional medicine with natural medicine.

Acid forming foods slowly create disease in your body. Alkaline forming foods slowly create healing in your body. – Garry Gordon

Juicing fruit and vegetables gives your body abundant enzymes, vitamins and minerals to supercharge your immune system and give you dynamic energy.

What you eat every day is creating your future health; aim for 80% alkaline forming foods and 20% acid forming foods to increase your longevity.

Your body is about 70% water; most fruit and vegetables are high water foods while cooked meat has very little water.

Gerson therapy: beetroot, apple and carrot juiced creates conditions in your body for healing many diseases.

Wheatgrass juice has mysterious healing qualities.

The more alkaline forming foods you eat like fruit and vegetables the more oxygen in your blood and the longer you shall live.

Fruit and vegetables were created by God, processed food was created by man. Who do you trust?

Let food be thy medicine. – Hippocrates

CHAPTER 2 – FITNESS

Exercise is the key not only to physical health but to peace of mind. – Nelson Mandela

For me, exercise is more than just physical, it's therapeutic. – Michelle Obama

Many exercise forms, aerobic exercise, yoga, weights, walking and more, have been shown to benefit mood. – Dr Andrew Weil

Those who think they have no time for exercise will sooner or later have to find time for illness. – Edward Stanley

Yoga allows you to find an inner peace that is not ruffled by the endless stresses and struggles of life. – B.K.S. Iyengar

Exercise should be regarded as a tribute to the heart. – Gene Tunney

Tai Chi – Balance, tranquillity and strength.

Life is like riding a wave. To keep your balance, you must keep moving. – Eric Carlson

Yoga is the fountain of youth. – Anonymous

All truly great thoughts are conceived by walking. – Friedrich Nietzsche

CHAPTER 3 – ATTITUDE

The game of life is a game of boomerangs. Our thoughts, deeds and words return to us sooner or later with astounding accuracy. – Florence Shinn

Surround yourself with people who can lift you higher. – Oprah

Where there is great love there are always miracles. – Willa Cather

When it rains look for rainbows. When it's dark look for stars.

Optimists look for opportunities in problems while pessimists look for problems in opportunities.

Because of the Law of Attraction, each of you is like a powerful magnet, attracting more of the way that you feel at any point in time. – Esther and Jerry Hicks

When you focus on gratitude, the universe sends you more things to be grateful for.

The universe has your back. – Gabby Bernstein

You just can't beat the person who never gives up. – Babe Ruth

It is time to live in the present moment and stop the past defining you.

The wound is the place where the light enters you. – Rumi

CHAPTER 4 – LIFE-LONG LEARNING

When you get out of your comfort zone that is where the real learning takes place.

A partner will bring up all your patterns. Don't avoid relationships, they are the best seminar in town. The truth is your partner is your guru. – Sondra Ray

Humility is the acceptance that someone can teach you something you don't know about yourself.

I have not failed. I have just found 10,000 ways that don't work. – Thomas A. Emerson

There is only one corner of the universe you can be certain of improving, and that's your own self. – Aldous Huxley

When we turn inwards, we surrender to the one and only truth, which is love. When we surrender to love, we can experience our darkest moment as the greatest catalyst for transformation. – Gabby Bernstein

In the silence of your heart you will slowly discover your purpose in life.

Learn to get in touch with the silence within yourself and know that everything in life has a purpose, there are no mistakes, no coincidences, all events are given to us as blessings, given to us to learn from. – Elizabeth Kubler Ross

Learning never exhausts the mind. – Leonardo da Vinci

CHAPTER 5 – DRINK PURE WATER

Pure water is the world's first and foremost medicine.

Water does not need preservatives, it comes from God.

Secrets of a waterfall, flow into the present moment and keep moving.

Many a headache is caused by dehydration, drink more pure water.

Tears are the safety valve of the body and they are composed of water.

Fruit and vegetables are about 70% water, your body is about 70% water and planet earth is about 70% water.

Benefits of drinking water: it helps you lose weight, it is a natural remedy for headaches, glowing skin, reduces your chances of getting sick, relieves fatigue, helps flush out toxins and help achieves greater longevity.

Pure water only comes in one flavour.

Just as a drop of water causes ripples in a pond, drinking pure water will cause ripples in your longevity.

Empty your mind, be formless, shapeless, like water. If you put water in a cup, it becomes the cup. You put water into a bottle and it becomes the bottle. You put it in a teapot it becomes a teapot. Now water can flow or it can crash into rocks by the sea. Be water my friend. – Bruce Lee

CHAPTER 6 – EATING FOODS WITH ABUNDANT ENZYMES

Natural yogurt is the elixir of longevity.

Sauerkraut tastes sour but it is sweet for building good bacteria in your colon.

Wheatgrass juice contains mystery enzymes that heal the body of diseases.

Kimchi is a spicy delight that brings the light of good bacteria to your colon.

Beetroot, apple and carrot juice to defeat disease with ease.

Juicing fruits and vegetables releases abundant enzymes, firing up your immune system and giving you abundant energy.

Sprouted grains are full of enzymes and B vitamins to defeat stress.

Kefir contains more good bacteria and enzymes than yogurt to lift your longevity and vitality.

Dandelion root tea is nature's way of cleaning your liver which is a powerhouse of enzyme activity.

As we grow older our bodies lose enzymes, let us grow younger by adding more enzymes.

CHAPTER 7 – AVOID STRESS

Let exercise be your stress reliever, not food.

Meditation is fasting for your mind and reduces stress.

It is time to focus on your blessings to build calmness and serenity and let go of what stresses you.

Diaphragm breathing will help reduce stress.

Today, I refuse to get stressed about things I cannot control or change.

Walking early in the morning heals the mind, body and spirit and in the silence you can sometimes hear the whispers of God.

It is time to let go of the past and focus on the present moment.

The worst things we imagine never seem to materialize.

Yoga is a way to find inner peace and calm.

A diamond is just a piece of charcoal that handled stress exceptionally well.

CHAPTER 8 – BALANCE

Balance is the key to the universe. – Hugh Grech

Life is like a bicycle, to keep balance, you must keep moving. – Albert Einstein

No person, no place and no thing has any power over us, for "we" are the only thinkers in our mind. When we create peace, harmony and balance in our minds, we will find it in our lives. – Louise Hay

Tolerance is the greatest gift of the mind, it requires the same effort of the brain that it takes to balance oneself on a bicycle. – Helen Keller

Beauty is only skin deep. I think what's really important is finding a balance of mind, body and spirit. – Jennifer Lopez

Love grounds you. It orients you. Love brings your awareness to others and yourself. Love opens your mind and heart to others and yourself. Love settles you and gives you balance. – Gary Zukav

We have seven faithful doctors: 1) Doctor love everybody, 2) Doctor forgiveness, 3) Doctor fruit, 4) Doctor vegetables, 5) Doctor pure water, 6) Doctor sunshine, and 7) Doctor exercise.

When there is balance between mind, body and spirit you will find peace.

CHAPTER 9 – FAMILY AND COMMUNITY

We are from many different countries and cultures but we were all created from the spirit of God.

Our family is our most important community.

The family is a circle of love and strength. Every obstacle faced together makes the circle stronger.

Join a community composed of your interests, that way you learn from them and they learn from you.

All cultures that have great longevity have a strong community that help each other in the spirit of sharing.

We can learn so much from the community of bees, sharing food, helping each other and making honey together.

Community is about sharing your knowledge so that your candle lights another candle and together we can spread more light.

A school and a university is a community of education where life-long learning is practiced.

A sporting community such as tennis, cricket, gym or baseball is a place to exercise your mind, body and spirit.

Let us be grateful to people who make us happy, they are the charming gardeners who make our souls blossom. – Marcel Proust

Love your family because there are three things that last forever, faith, hope and love, but the greatest is love.

CHAPTER 10 – SPIRIT

Affirmation prayer: I am the light in the darkness. I am the love in the hate. I am the calmness in the storm. I am the courage in the hate. – Gordana Biernat

See the light in others and treat them as if that is all you see. – Dr Wayne Dyer

When faced with challenges, God may close one door but will always open another door. – Author unknown

Trees grown in silence, the moon, the sun, and the stars move in silence. God is a friend of silence. – Author unknown

Faith is the daring of the soul to go further than it can see. – William Newton Clarke

Let my candle light your candle and together we can spread more light. – Garry Gordon

When you begin to dance with the energy of the universe, your life flows naturally, incredible synchronicity presents itself, creative solutions abound. – Gabby Bernstein

After the storm, the rainbow comes out. – Annierose

Printed in the United States
By Bookmasters